emily kelly's
commonsense

Pilates

simple
techniques for
a strong, *lithe*
healthier body

emily kelly's
commonsense

Pilates

photography by **christine hanscomb** and **stephen swain**

LORENZ BOOKS

First published in 2000 by Lorenz Books

Lorenz Books is an imprint of
Anness Publishing Limited
Hermes House
88–89 Blackfriars Road
London SE1 8HA
www.lorenzbooks.com

© Anness Publishing Limited 2001

Published in the USA by Lorenz Books,
Anness Publishing Inc., 27 West 20th Street,
New York, NY 10011

This edition distributed in Canada by
Raincoast Books
8680 Cambie Street
Vancouver   British Columbia V6P 6M9

A CIP catalogue record for this book is available
from the British Library

Publisher: **Joanna Lorenz**
Project Editor: **Debra Mayhew**
Designer: **Lisa Tai**
Photography: **Christine Hanscomb** (colour)
and **Stephen Swain** (black and white)
Production Controller: **Don Campaniello**
Editorial reader: **Diane Ashmore**
Illustrator: **David Cook, Linden Artists**

10 9 8 7 6 5 4 3 2 1

Publisher's note: The reader should not regard the
recommendations, ideas and techniques expressed
and described in this book as substitutes for the advice
of a qualified medical practitioner or other qualified
professional. Any use to which the recommendations,
ideas and techniques are put is at the reader's sole
discretion and risk.

Contents

author's note

My aim in writing this book is to guide you through the Pilates technique in a stress-free and accessible way. I have always felt a huge passion for movement and exercise, and what I now hope to do is pass on some of that enthusiasm and energy to you.

When I started working as a fitness teacher, I tried to respond to my clients' individual needs by looking at all available types of activity and took courses in Alexander Technique, resistance training, swimming, circuit training, kick-boxing, boxercise, fitness assessment training, ante- and postnatal training, exercise to music, Indian champissage (head massage), self-defence, yoga and exercise counselling. I even tried line dancing!

I finally discovered Pilates after a visit from an American relative who had the perfect dancer's body: long and lean with fantastic elegance and posture. I endeavoured to find out everything I could about this technique so I took classes, studied and practised. To me, it was like "coming home": the moves were graceful

△ Regular Pilates practice helped me to correct muscular imbalances, made me stronger and leaner and reduced my risk of injury.

Emily Kelly

and challenging and reminded me of the time I had spent doing ballet and gymnastics. I felt I was being taken back to basics and I loved the attention to alignment and the focus.

I became obsessed: every client had to try Pilates, and the results spoke for themselves. Everyone commented on the dramatic difference to their appearance, finding that their spine felt flexible and strong and their abdominals became flatter and tauter. Changes in posture brought about a more confident, slimmer appearance. What struck me as a teacher was how much people enjoyed Pilates, even the completely exercise-phobic. At whatever point you are starting, stick to this programme and your body will change, and this will have a balancing effect on your life. I wish you every success.

introducing
Pilates

In this first chapter we look at who can benefit from regular Pilates practice, why this book is different, and, most importantly, what you can expect to achieve. Refer to this chapter again when you feel that you need any additional motivation ...

If you have tried other exercise programmes in the past and wondered why their success has been limited, find out why Pilates is different and why its practice will become an essential, and enjoyable, part of your life.

introduction

Why another exercise book? What is it about Pilates that makes it such a favourite in gyms and dance schools and such a respected and popular activity? With all the different exercise videos and books on the market, what makes this book special?

Maybe the answer is in the book's title: commonsense. This book is designed to be an accessible manual that you can integrate into your life. It explains the key elements of Pilates and takes you by the hand through a comprehensive range of exercises. The programme aims to be very user-friendly: it is designed for beginners to Pilates but more advanced variations of many exercises are included so that you can set yourself a greater challenge as you progress.

The "first position" in each exercise is the most basic option. If you are new to Pilates then always start with this one, otherwise you will not have mastered the control and the focus needed to perform the exercise correctly. During a Pilates session your main concern should be the feeling that you get from doing the movement correctly, not how many repetitions you can do. The

△ Pilates combines stretches and strengthening exercises, making it one of the safest and most effective forms of exercise.

△ Pilates help to re-define posture, creating a relaxed, confident stance. It is worth remembering that the correct posture can give an illusion of a 6 lb weight loss.

"second position" should only be attemped after you have a clear understanding of the first position. For some people this may take two or more months. For others, it may take as little as three weeks. Everyone is different. It is not a competition, just progress at your own rate. The "third position" is a more intense variation still.

You may find that you progress faster with some exercises than with others. This is perfectly normal. For example, you may have a slight imbalance in your body that is being strongly challenged by the movement. Have faith in your knowledge of how your own body feels.

The holistic approach

This book aims to get you to look at exercise in a holistic way and to help you integrate it into your daily life with only minimal

disturbance. It does not set out to turn you into an Olympic athlete. It might, however, give you that little push you need to start exercising by explaining just why it is important, not just for aesthetic purposes but to help you avoid pain and injury, to make you feel good about your body and to increase your self-esteem.

The intention is that you will find the programme clear, logical and simple to remember, so that it will be quite easy to make it a regular part of your daily routine – just like brushing your teeth – because exercise really should be a matter of course. It's just common sense. You need to take care of your body at least as well as you take care of your car. You probably expect your car to last you six or seven years, and oil changes, tune-ups and wheel alignments are common practice for every car owner. How long do you want your body to last you?

Everyone can benefit

So who can benefit from this programme? Basically, Pilates has something to offer everyone, whatever your age or current fitness level. Although you will get stronger all over, one of the main benefits of Pilates is an increase in core strength. This is a phrase that is used over and over again in connection with Pilates, and it refers to the important abdominal and back muscles at your centre that support your whole body whether moving or at rest. As these muscles are strengthened, your posture will improve and you will find it easier to go about your daily tasks.

If you are completely new to Pilates, you will find these exercises different from others you may have tried. First of all, Pilates is a series of movements that flow into one another without pauses. Most conventional exercise starts and stops: you might do 12 repetitions of a move, rest, and then start up again with the next sequence. Pilates concentrates on the body as a whole, stretching some muscles, strengthening

▷ Pilates creates a strong, lean, balanced body. This reduces the risk of injury and helps to elimate nagging aches and pains.

others and, by helping you to function more effectively, reducing the risk of injury, not only while you are exercising but in everything you do.

Many people who take up Pilates are pleased to discover that only a small number of repetitions are needed per exercise in comparison with other conventional methods. If you are performing the movements correctly, up to ten repetitions will be more than adequate. This means that you can give each repetition your full effort and concentration: you will be maximizing the potential of the exercise without growing tired or bored with continual repetitions.

The importance of focus

Another distinguishing feature of Pilates is that to practise it you must be totally focused and concentrated, and this concentration creates a mind-body connection. This doesn't mean that conventional exercise can be done without thought of course, but it does mean that Pilates needs all your attention and focus in order to get the best results. If you sometimes feel overwhelmed by everyday problems and stresses, giving all your attention to the

movements of a Pilates sequence can help to still the insistent clamour of your daily life, acting like meditation to calm your mind and help you see things more clearly. This total concentration and attention to alignment and detail makes Pilates quite unique and very satisfying.

Be kind to yourself

When you start the programme, it is important that you do not place any expectations on yourself. Pilates is about the feeling you

are getting from the exercise, not about how many repetitions you can do, how long you exercise for or how many advanced exercises you can work through. Some of the movements are very subtle and to an observer it may appear that you are doing very little. You should check throughout the exercises that

▽ Within weeks of beginning regular Pilates practice, you will see a clear improvement. Pilates creates long, lean muscles with no risk of developing a bulky, overdeveloped physique.

▷

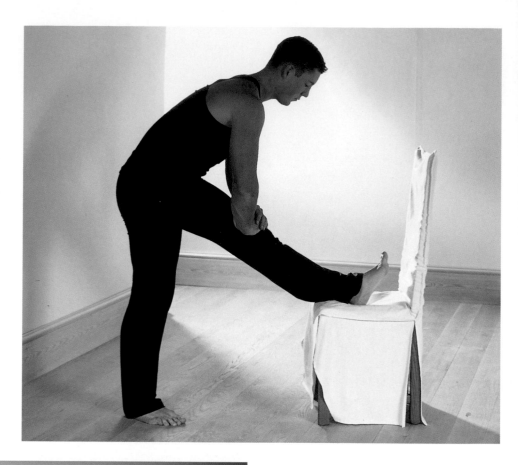

▷ Pilates should be combined with healthy
eating and regular cardiovascular exercise
for optimum results.

out the exercises that your spine is in neutral (unless otherwise stated), that the abdominals are contracted, that you are not holding your breath at any time, that the muscles not involved in the movement are relaxed (it is common to hold tension in the jaw and shoulders), and that the movements are controlled. All these factors are the key elements that make Pilates so effective, and they are fully explained on the following pages.

Pilates is a very personal experience. Listen to your body and stop if anything feels uncomfortable or causes pain – though this should not be confused with an exercise being challenging. It could be that a particular exercise is not right for you at this time; you can always come back to it on another occasion, or try the less intense version of the same exercise. If you simply cannot focus on an exercise during a session, choose another exercise from the same category; don't waste your time and create negative feeling for a movement.

The endorphin effect

You will sometimes hear regular exercisers talking about the high they get from activity: what they are describing is the production of endorphins, chemicals in the brain that are stimulated by exercise and have similar effects to that of opiates. If you need any more encouragement to get started, consider this: tests have shown that people who suffer from illness and depression are significantly helped by taking exercise.

As well as describing each exercise in detail, the book gives advice on putting together a sequence to help you achieve the benefits you are seeking, and on incorporating Pilates into an all-round fitness regime of exercise and healthy eating. Start investing in the present and future health of your body, today.

◁ Regular practice of Pilates will help you
achieve a long, lean, strong physique.

The history of Pilates

Recently it has become almost impossible to open a magazine and not find mention of a Pilates-based exercise programme. Everyone is talking about this "new" form of exercise, especially having seen the way it has sculpted celebrities such as Courtney Love, Sophie Dahl, Madonna and Melanie Griffiths. We jogged in the 70s, did aerobics with Jane Fonda in the 80s, took up weight-training in the 90s; in the new millennium we are discovering the mind-body experience.

In reality, Pilates has been around for a century. For ballet dancers, it has been a well-kept secret as the perfect way to become strong and centred without building bulk. Only in the past few years has the fitness world embraced Pilates, and this accounts for its sudden and well-deserved popularity as a form of exercise.

Joseph Pilates was born in Germany in 1880. He was a sickly child and suffered from asthma, rickets and rheumatic fever, which left him with a burning desire to become physically stronger. By the age of 14 he was an avid body-builder with a well-sculpted physique. He practised all types of sports, such as skiing, diving and gymnastics. At 32 he moved to England, where he made his living as a boxer, circus performer and self-defence instructor for detectives.

◁ The Pilates method was originally developed to build strength and increase immunity to disease. Today, the many modified forms of the techniques still teach your body to work at its most efficient.

13

introducing Pilates

When World War I broke out Pilates was interned in the Isle of Man. Being such a keen fan of exercise, Pilates decided that his fellow internees should get fit under his training. His efforts paid off, as none of his trainees succumbed to the massive influenza epidemic that killed millions after the war. He also worked as a hospital orderly, encountering many war casualties. He started working with some of the disabled patients, using his own body weight to move their limbs and devising special equipment to aid their progress. This consisted of springs attached to their hospital beds which gave gentle resistance to aid muscle strengthening and stretching: these were the prototypes of the machines that are used today.

Pilates believed that imbalances in the body and habitual patterns of movement cause injuries. He observed the links between weak areas of the body and over-

compensation (if you are weak in one area the rest of the body has to support the imbalance), and the exercises he devised were based around re-education and the re-alignment of the body.

In 1926 Pilates and his wife Clara moved to New York where they set up an exercise studio. By 1940 the dance community had become aware of his fitness programmes, including George Balanchine and other members of the New York City Ballet.

Pilates had a number of students who went on to set up their own studios and so the method spread, each teacher adding their own personal twists, as they continue to do today. It would be rare to find two instructors who teach Pilates in exactly the same way.

Since Pilates' death, followers of his methods have modified the original 34 exercises and made them more user-friendly. The Pilates method is practised in one of two ways: using equipment called a re-former, an updated version of the original springs, or as free body exercises using only a mat. The latter is the version that you will be taught in this book.

◁ Performing artists, such as singers, dancers, actors and models have long used Pilates' methods to improve posture, align their body, gain strength and avoid injury.

The benefits of Pilates

Muscles can be divided into two groups: prime movers and postural. The prime movers are those muscles involved in movement, such as the hamstrings at the back of the thighs or the deltoids in the shoulders. Postural muscles, such as the deep abdominal muscle called the transverse abdominis, work to maintain stability. This core stability is essential when the body is moving, for example, when creating a firm platform for keeping the pelvis still while running, or controlling the position of the shoulder blade while throwing.

Muscle imbalances can occur through repetitive strain or faulty mechanics, and result in an uneven pull of the muscles around a joint. This imbalance may eventually cause injury to that joint. The pain that results will inhibit the postural or stabilizing muscles around the joint and, as a result, these muscles weaken, making the injured joint even more unstable and still more susceptible to further injury and pain. And so the cycle repeats. Even when the area is no longer painful, these muscles do not automatically strengthen again. This is why injuries tend to re-occur. To recover fully from injury, the muscles in that area need to be specifically strengthened and their co-ordination retrained again.

Trunk or core stability requires strength, endurance and co-ordination of the stabilizing abdominal, pelvic floor and lower back muscles. Stability is necessary to

▽ **The anterior and posterior views of the human muscular system show the main muscles of the front and back of the body. Although this is a simple diagram only, it will help you to gain a clear understanding of the location of the muscles used throughout your Pilates practice. Be aware, though, that Pilates uses many other supporting muscle groups during different phases of a movement.**

THE MUSCULAR SYSTEM

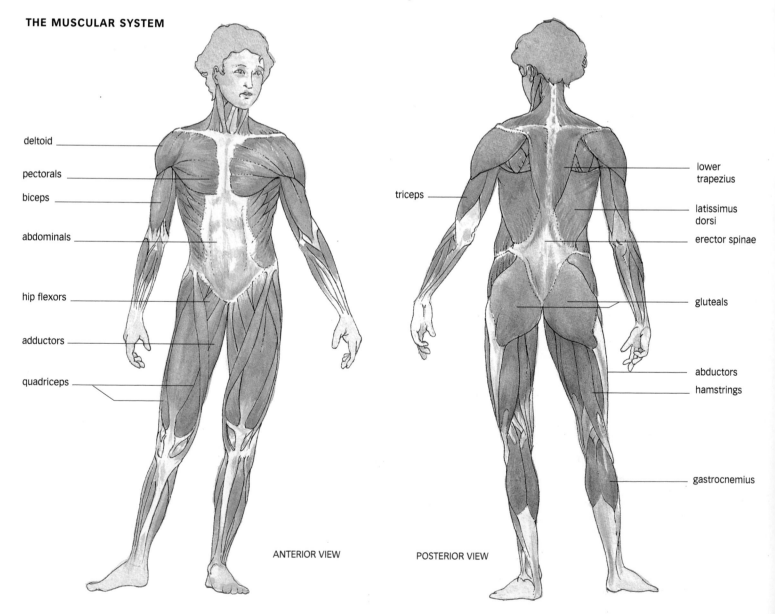

deltoid

pectorals

biceps

abdominals

hip flexors

adductors

quadriceps

triceps

lower trapezius

latissimus dorsi

erector spinae

gluteals

abductors

hamstrings

gastrocnemius

ANTERIOR VIEW   POSTERIOR VIEW

◁ **Throughout the day try to give yourself a posture bodycheck. Try to pinpoint your bad habits as awareness is half the battle.**

more energy, extra alertness during waking hours and a general sense of well-being.

For the more experienced exerciser, Pilates can help to highlight imbalances throughout the body. The attention to detail and the concentration given to the movements can challenge even elite professional athletes, who often comment that they feel like beginners again after trying it. What appear to be the simplest of movements can be incredibly challenging when performed correctly, so do not worry if even the first position of an exercise seems hard to you: in terms of Pilates this is a good thing. As long as you work at your own pace, paying attention to how your body feels during the movement, Pilates is perfectly safe and very effective.

support and protect the lower back from injury, to help with general postural alignment and to allow the release of the hips for greater freedom of movement. Better core stability can therefore reduce the chance of injury. Improving it is often the way finally to get rid of niggling back problems that you may have suffered from for years. Core stability exercises are an important part of the Pilates method, which focuses on improving the strength and control of these stabilizing muscles.

The Pilates programme is very enjoyable and you should soon feel results which will motivate you to continue. If you adhere to it, you will be rewarded by improved posture, an enhanced feeling of balance, reduction in aches, pains and stiffness, greater flexibility and a longer, leaner, more highly toned body. As your posture improves, you will look as if you have lost weight, and one of the most frequently heard comments from people who are new to Pilates is that they feel "as if they have grown". This is because they have learned to lengthen up through the spine to its maximum potential, making them look slimmer and feel more confident.

Regular Pilates sessions will help your co-ordination and enhance your balance, which is of special importance through the

aging process. You will gain strength in a balanced way, so that tight, tense areas are stretched and weak ones strengthened. The realignment of your body will also make it easier for you to use it correctly. You will feel more relaxed and less stressed and will possibly benefit from other "by-products" such as more refreshing sleep,

▷ **Many osteopaths recommend Pilates to aid recovery and rehabilitation as well as a way of preventing possible imbalances or injuries. Remember though, if you feel pain or have an existing injury, always check with a medical professional before starting a new exercise programme.**

PILATES AND OSTEOPATHY

My introduction to Pilates followed a serious back injury. I was eager to recover as quickly as possible, and for the injury not to recur. I am a competitive runner (a former International 400m runner), so I did not want the injury to affect my training. I found a class and was impressed by the specificity of the exercises and how much more stable my back felt after several weeks of regular sessions. Since maintaining a regular regime, my back has felt better and my sports performance has improved. I now incorporate clinically based Pilates exercises into the rehabilitation of my patients and recommend it to them as an excellent way to improve their own stability.

Alex Fugallo
DO, ND, Bsc (Hons) Osteopathic Medicine
Registered Osteopath

The exercise environment

It is important to "set the stage" for your Pilates routine, creating a serene environment that will not divert you from the mind-body connection. So, before you begin, block out any distractions and ensure that your exercise session will not be interrupted. Here are a few tips for preparing your exercise environment:

• Find a comfortable, quiet area to work in, where you will have enough room to lie down without hitting your head on the coffee table.

• Turn off your phone, the television and any other machines that might disturb your routine.

• Aim to create gentle lighting, using natural daylight if possible or a soft lamp.

• Burning essential oils can help to create the right atmosphere: try lavender if you want a relaxing, calming session or orange to uplift or invigorate. Lemon is refreshing and is said to aid concentration: simply experiment to see what suits you.

• It is important to use a good exercise mat. Look for one that will protect your spine when you lie down; it should be firm but have enough padding so you can't feel the floor. Make sure it is non-slip and long enough for you to lie on when you are completely stretched out.

• Wear comfortable clothes; cotton is best. Avoid tight elastic bands, but do not wear very baggy clothes: you will feel stronger and sleeker in contoured clothes which allow you to move and stretch freely.

• Listen to soft, relaxing music with no harsh sounds. New age or classical music works well. Alternatively, a recording of natural sounds or crashing waves might be a good choice.

• Try not to have a heavy meal before starting exercise of any kind. Digesting the food while you are trying to work your muscles could cause cramps or indigestion. Allow at least two hours after a main meal before exercising. If you are hungry before you exercise eat a piece of fruit to tide you over.

▽ **Create a spacious and comfortable area for practising Pilates. Remove any distractions so that you will not be disturbed and wear comfortable, streamlined clothes so that you feel in tune with your body throughout.**

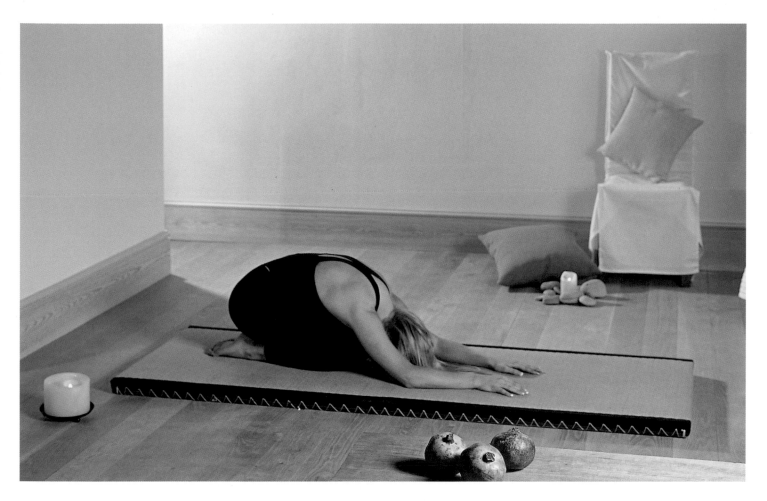

It is important to be well hydrated at all times – especially when exercising. Always have a bottle of water to hand and take small sips throughout the session. Drink water before and after exercise, and try to get into the habit of always having water with you.

△ Using gentle lighting helps to set a calm mood especially during the relaxation phases of your workout. Scented candles can be very calming, try fresh sea scents.

• A sports drink is only necessary if you will be exercising strenuously for 90 minutes or more. Sports drinks replenish lost electrolytes (these are sodium, potassium and chloride) but this is not a problem unless you sweat excessively during an extended bout of exercise .

• Pilates is done barefoot, so do not worry about trainers or socks. This helps you to judge more accurately the distribution of weight in your feet as you exercise.

• Before you start your Pilates session spend a couple of minutes (longer if it is possible) focusing on how your body feels. Do you feel tension in any specific area or are you stiff or tight in certain muscles? Be your own fitness advisor and tailor your routine around your body's needs. For example, if you feel stiff then you may choose to add more stretches into your programme for that day for a better workout.

△ Try to drink a little before and after your Pilates session, and take sips whilst you exercise. Water is the best drink. Not only does it keep you hydrated but you will have the added benefit of glowing skin.

• You know your body better than anyone else does. Be aware that your body's needs change daily and try to respond to those needs. Be prepared to adjust your routine in order to gain maximum benefit from your programme. But take care to keep your routine balanced so that you are not just doing the exercises you find easy.

△ Pilates is performed barefoot. You could paint your toenails so that you feel beautiful while working out.

Key elements of Pilates

Some concepts are referred to repeatedly in Pilates: these are the "key elements" that make it more than just a sequence of movements. Keep them in mind throughout your sessions, relating them to each exercise, and as you become more familiar with the technique they will start to make more sense to you. They will help you to get the most benefit from each movement, and also keep the exercises safe and comfortable. Some of these key elements will come more naturally to you than others, but do not feel discouraged. They will eventually become automatic and you will find yourself applying the same principles to other forms of activity, because they are based on attention to detail and alignment, safety and commonsense.

breathing

Breathing is something you do unconsciously, but when you are relaxed and calm your breathing pattern is different from when you are tense, anxious or negative.

At times of tension and stress, breathing is usually irregular and shallow, and does not completely fulfil your need for oxygen. If you learn to control your breathing while practising Pilates as well as during daily activity, it will help you to maintain your energy and stay relaxed.

Holding your breath causes tension in your muscles, which decreases when you exhale. For this reason, athletes learn to exhale when executing certain movements such as a tennis serve, a basketball dunk or a golf swing: they are programmed to exhale on the maximum effort. In sports that require a maximum effort during a longer period of time, such as power-lifting, elite athletes will hold their breath. This gives their muscles added stability but has several potentially negative effects on their blood pressure. Remember that these athletes are aiming at a particular goal: they want to win medals at all costs, sometimes even by endangering their health. You should never

hold your breath when exercising. In Pilates, it is sometimes difficult to gauge which of the movements is the one that takes maximum effort. Most of the movements maintain tension in the torso at all times, but your breathing should always be regular and relaxed.

When starting out on this or any other exercise programme, strive to master the general movement first, then focus on the breathing patterns. It is often the case that correct breathing patterns start to come naturally as the body tries to help itself, but you can practise breathing control exercises when you are not moving to help you learn the correct technique. During the exercises try not to let the ribs flare up (push upwards and outwards away from your spine), which sometimes goes hand in hand with arching the spine. Aim to keep the ribs the same distance from your hips, just sliding them out to the sides and then back again as you breathe. This is described as breathing laterally.

Breathing exercise

Here is a simple breath control strategy that you can practise at any time. Regulating your breathing will enhance your body awareness and control and make you feel calm and centred.

△ **1** Place your hands with your palms under your chest, on your ribs, and your fingers loosely interlocked. Inhale slowly and continuously through your nose, to a count of four. Do not strain, keep yourself relaxed.

△ **2** As you inhale concentrate on allowing your ribs to expand laterally: your fingers should gently part. Don't let your ribs jut forward. Exhale slowly, expelling all the breath from your lungs, then repeat.

◁ During your Pilates session you must give each movement your full concentration. Really focus and *feel* the muscles working.

▷ If you do not feel in complete control of a movement, then try a less intense version. Return to the more advanced variation at a later date.

concentration

Your muscles respond better to a training stimulus if the brain is concentrated on the effort. Remember that it is the brain that sends out the signal to the muscle to contract. So, it is imperative that you concentrate on the work you expect the muscle to perform.

It is very easy to get distracted while exercising if you do not set the right mood, avoiding intrusive sounds or disturbances that will take your mind off what you are doing. It is also necessary to prepare yourself mentally to focus on your body and the work that it will be doing.

control

All movements should be performed slowly and with absolute control. The faster you do anything, the less actual muscle mass you will use to do the exercise: instead, you will be

▽ Try to begin and end each session with a few moments of complete relaxation.

using momentum. Most Pilates movements are not static; they should be continuous but at the same time controlled and precise.

flow

Pilates movements cannot be likened to repetitions of a conventional exercise. They are continuous. Try to "link" one movement with the next, maintaining a steady flow of energy

△ Maintain a steady flow of energy, keeping movements graceful and fluid.

throughout the session. You will not be stopping and starting as in conventional exercise, but flowing like a steadily turning wheel.

relaxation

Pilates is a gradual re-education of the body, and in order to benefit from it you must try not to create unnecessary tension. This would eventually create an imbalance in the body, which is the very thing you are trying to remedy. Watch especially for tension in the neck and jaw, but you may hold it anywhere – even in the feet. During a session, give yourself little mental checks from head to toe and you will start to see where you tend to hold tension. Awareness is half the battle.

adherence

No exercise programme works unless you do it! Adopt this programme as part of your life and make it as much part of your daily routine as brushing your teeth: physical activity is as much a way of taking care of your body as personal hygiene.

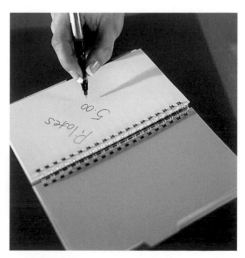

△ Pilates practice must be consistent in order for you to see and feel the benefits.

Core strength

The principal aim of the exercises is to create core strength, which will be the powerhouse for the rest of your body. When you reach a level of understanding of core strength Pilates starts to feel like an altogether different form of exercise: you begin to get a feel for your body working as a whole in a very focused, concentrated way.

The abdominals and back form the centre of the body, from which all movements in Pilates are initiated. If you look at a ferris wheel in a funfair, there is movement around the wheel but the powerhouse is the centre because everything is controlled from there. This is how you should view your body. Your centre should be your first priority, because without sufficient strength in this area you are vulnerable to injury. So, what are these muscles and how do you locate them?

▷ The illustration displays the key abdominal muscles used in Pilates. These are the muscles used when we refer to "working from a strong centre" or developing "core strength".

rectus abdominis

transverse abdominis

internal abdominal obliques

external abdominal oblique

muscles that stabilize the torso

Rectus abdominis: This is a wide and long muscle that runs all the way down from the sternum (breast bone) to the pubic bone. The rectus abdominis helps to maintain correct posture and allows forward flexion.

Obliques: These are located at the waist, and there are actually two sets: the internal and external obliques. They allow you to rotate at the waist as well as flexing laterally (to illustrate this, imagine that you are picking up a suitcase by your side).

Transverse abdominis: This muscle is located behind the rectus abdominis, like a "girdle" wrapped around your stomach. It is used when you draw your navel towards your spine, and is the muscle that contracts when you cough.

building core strength

By stabilizing the torso you are creating a "co-contraction" between the abdominal muscles and the back muscles. This means that all these muscles are working together to create a stable entity. In most people they are weak, and in the back they can be tense and tight. In this situation the spine may be pulled out of alignment, causing improper posture and risk of injury. When the back muscles and the abdominals are strong and flexible it becomes easier to maintain correct posture. Pilates strengthens and stretches these core muscles, helping to correct imbalances and reducing the chances of suffering back pain.

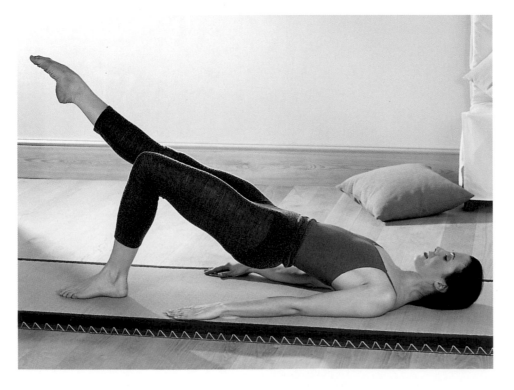

◁ Pilates exercises are designed to build up your core strength.

Locating the transverse abdominis

Sit or stand upright, inhale and pull your stomach towards your back, imagining that you are wearing very tight jeans and trying to pull your tummy away from the waistband. This is what you will be doing during all the Pilates exercises.

△ **1** Lie on your tummy with your head relaxed and supported on your folded hands or on a small cushion under your forehead. Keep your head in alignment with your back and the back of your neck long, without shortening the front. Try to keep your hip bones on the floor and relax your shoulders.

△ **2** Inhale, then as you exhale pull your navel towards your spine, trying to create an arch under your abdominals. You may not be able to lift very far up at first: this is not important as long as you understand the concept. Gently lift your shoulders back and draw your shoulder blades down your spine.

△ If sliding your shoulder blades down your spine is a baffling request, practise this subtle movement by standing up with your arms by your sides. Keeping your back straight, push your fingertips towards the floor. Do not force your arms down or lock them into position. Try to keep the shoulder blades close to the back of the ribcage. This is very useful for limiting tension around the shoulders, which tends to make you pull your shoulders up to your ears.

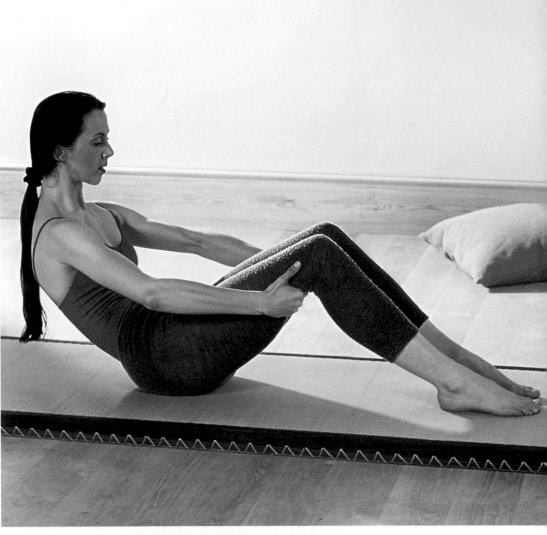

△ Every movement should be controlled via your abdominals. Keep bringing your attention and focus back to pulling your navel towards your spine.

Neutral spine

A healthy spine has natural curves that should be preserved and respected but not exaggerated. The term "neutral spine" refers to the natural alignment of the spine. If you have any serious pain in your back, check with a physician before embarking on any exercise programme. The main curves are:

1 **The cervical spine**: the area behind the head, along the back of the neck, is concave; it should curve gently inwards.

2 **The thoracic vertebrae**: the largest area of the back curves very slightly outwards.

3 **The lumbar spine**: the lower back should curve slightly inwards; it should not be flat or over curved.

4 **The sacral spine**: the sacral curve is at the bottom of your spine and curves gently outwards.

It is important to allow the spine to rest in its natural position to prevent stresses and imbalances. During Pilates movements you

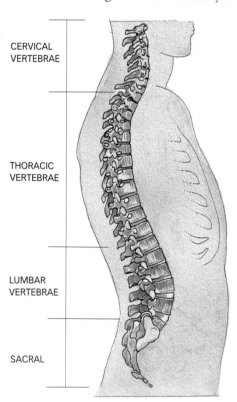

CERVICAL
VERTEBRAE

THORACIC
VERTEBRAE

LUMBAR
VERTEBRAE

SACRAL

Finding neutral spine

The importance of neutral spine cannot be emphasized enough, as it allows your spine to elongate and relax. Before starting an exercise it can be helpful to roll gently between the two extreme positions and then try to fall comfortably between the two.

◁ **1** Tilt your pelvis, flattening your back into the floor.

◁ **2** Tilt your pelvis in the opposite direction, creating an arch under your lower back. Make this movement slow and take care not to hold for too long or you may cause tension in your lower spine.

◁ **3** Find a position between these two extremes in which your back feels natural and comfortable: this is neutral spine. Unless otherwise stated, you should always work from this position during your Pilates routine.

should ensure (unless otherwise directed) that your back is not flat or pushed into the floor, although this can be tempting in order to achieve a flatter tummy. What you tend to do in this position is grip at the hip flexors (the muscles located at the top of the thighs) thus creating tension in a place that is commonly tight anyway. You must also try to avoid over curving your spine, as this pushes the abdominals forwards and tightens the muscles around the spine. "Neutral spine" lies in between these two extremes and echoes the natural and safe position that your spine prefers.

◁ **The diagram shows the four natural spinal curves. These curves help to cushion some of the shock from our daily activities – even walking creates some mild stress. One of the key elements of Pilates is the close attention given to the alignment of the spine during all movements.**

Pelvic floor muscles

The pelvic floor muscles act as a dynamic platform at the base of the pelvis, functioning both as a support mechanism and as an aid to bowel and bladder function. Well-trained pelvic floor muscles may also improve orgasmic potential in women and erectile function in men.

Pelvic floor muscle activity is a "lift and squeeze" movement: it is the action used to stop midstream urine flow and to stop the passage of wind. It is essential to perform this movement accurately in order to improve the muscles. A woman can tell if she is using the correct muscles by examining herself with a mirror. During a pelvic floor muscle contraction she should see an anal squeeze and an upward movement of her perineum. Inside the vagina, she or her partner should be able to feel a vaginal pressure. A man should see an anal squeeze with the penis lifting at the same time.

Once you have found the correct movement, the next part of the strengthening process is to hold the contraction and to repeat it. At first, you may be able to perform only short holds, but the aim is eventually to hold each contraction for ten seconds. The number of times that you repeat the contraction also depends on your ability; the aim is eventually to repeat the hold ten times.

As well as these sustained holds, you should also practise short, sharp, fast contractions, again in sets of ten. To strengthen the muscles you will need to exercise them up to six times a day. To maintain the resulting change you should remember to exercise them to their full ability at least once a day.

As the brain controls the action of muscles in groups rather than individually, it is important when exercising to consider those muscles that work well together. It is now believed that the pelvic floor muscles work best in conjunction with the transverse abdominis, which is contracted constantly during Pilates exercises. Once you are familiar with Pilates movements you can add pelvic floor muscle lifting and squeezing as you contract your abdominals.

Jeanette Haslam
MPhil, MSCP, SRP

▷ **The pelvic floor muscles are often ignored but are important to exercise. For maximum benefit, especially for women who have had children, the exercises should be performed daily.**

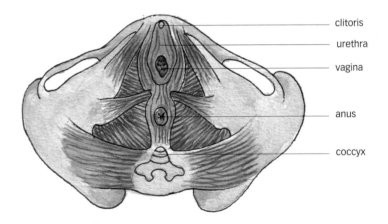

clitoris
urethra
vagina
anus
coccyx

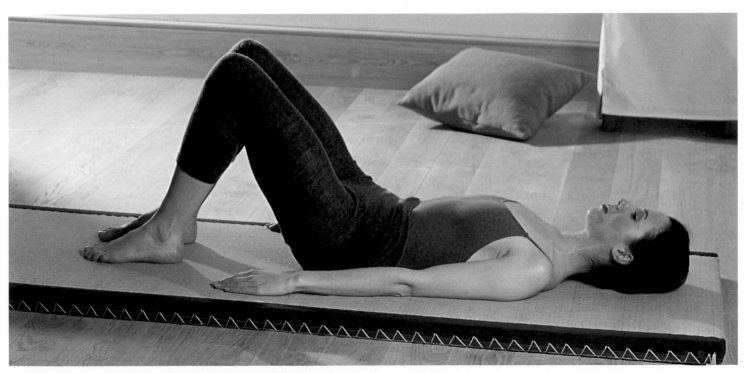

△ **When you become more familiar with Pilates, try adding pelvic floor contractions as you exercise.**

warming up and mobility exercises

This chapter is dedicated to preparing

the body for the demands we are going

to make on it. One of the benefits of

warm-up exercises is the release of fluids

into the joints making the muscles more

pliable, reducing the risk of injury as well

as making muscular responses faster and

more precise. By regularly practising

mobilizing exercises, you decrease your

risk of sustaining injuries when exercising

and make even everyday activities easier

to perform.

Exercises for warming-up

The first part of any exercise routine should be a warm-up to raise the core temperature of your muscles. If you pull a cold elastic band too hard it snaps, but once it is warm it becomes more pliable and will stretch further. The same applies to your muscles. The warm-up prepares you psychologically for activity, getting you in the mood. It also increases the efficiency of the neuromuscular pathways, thus speeding up the signals sent from the brain to your muscles.

Keep your movements flowing and gentle during the warm-up: do not force your body or overstretch. Adopt the correct breathing patterns each time and keep the spine in neutral. Repeat each of the warm-up exercises five times.

Perform all exercises with flow and complete concentration. Work from a strong centre and avoid holding on to any unnecessary tension. Breathe wide and full.

Arm crosses

These are great for warming up the shoulders and upper back. The movement should be continuous and flowing: think of the graceful way in which a ballet dancer's arms move. As you do the exercise, watch for tension in the neck; your spine should stay in neutral and your abdominals hollowed. Imagine you are trying to reach both sides of the room and lengthen out through your arms and up through your spine.

△**1** Stand with your feet about hip-width apart and cross one hand in front of the other. Relax your shoulders and lengthen up through your spine, keeping your head in alignment.

△**2** Inhale to prepare and, as you exhale, take your arms out to the sides, palms up. Keep your shoulders relaxed and slide your shoulder blades down your spine as you lift your arms. Lower your arms to begin again. This should be performed at a moderately fast pace but should always be controlled and flowing.

Shoulder circles

A good way to relieve tension in the shoulders and upper back, this exercise also mobilizes the shoulders. It is a movement that many people tend to stumble on naturally when they are feeling stiff. Make the movement slow and controlled, breathing in wide and full through the ribs. Keep the spine in neutral.

△1 Stand with your feet hip-width apart, lengthen up through your spine and do not let the abdominals sag. Inhale to prepare. As you exhale, roll your shoulders forwards up to your ears and then around.

△ 2 Concentrate on trying to form a complete circle. Think about the shape you are making: is it a circle or an egg-shape? Create as big a circle as you can in one direction then the other.

Arm sweeps

This big, sweeping movement will wake you up and help with a "fuzzy head". It also mobilizes the spine, lower body and shoulders. Try to move in a fluid, rhythmic way at a constant speed.

△1 Stand with your feet close together, knees and shoulders relaxed, keep the abdominals hollowed. Extend your arms overhead and lengthen up through the spine while keeping your feet flat on the floor and your head in alignment.

△ 2 Inhale to prepare, then drop your chin to your chest and roll down through your spine, letting your arms flow behind you.

△ 3 Bend your knees as your arms sweep back and again as you bring them forward and up over your head to begin again, lengthening up through your spine as you return to standing.

▷

Walking through the feet

You may be surprised at how stiff your feet and ankles get, and this exercise is designed to wake up the feet, ankles and calves. It's a good idea to warn them gently of the activity to come, so that they provide a strong, secure base.

◁ From standing, lift the heel on one foot then the other in a natural walking movement, bending the knees. Keep the spine in neutral and the abdominals hollowed. Keep this movement rhythmic and continuous, always lengthening up through the spine.

Standing balance

This is a more advanced way to warm up the feet and lower legs, which may also challenge your balance. Try to keep your weight central and concentrate on each part of your foot as you rise and come back down on to your heels. This movement is performed at a moderately slow pace.

◁ Stand with your feet hip-width apart and make sure that your toes are not clenched but relaxed. Keep your spine in neutral, abdominals hollowed, and place your hands on your hips to help you balance. Keeping your head in alignment, come all the way up on to your toes. Hold the balance for a few seconds, then lower your heels slowly to begin again.

Relaxation position

This is not a movement, just a comfortable position. Try always to start and end your Pilates sessions with a couple of minutes in the relaxation position. It will help you focus and get in contact with your body, as well as making you feel relaxed and refreshed. Concentrate on each area of your body, from your head down, and try to observe any tension, particularly in your jaw and face, shoulders and hips. Some people even clench their feet. Just notice where your areas of tension are and gently focus on relaxing. Try to visualize your spine lengthening and sinking into the floor. Imagine you are lying on warm sand and let it support your spine. This position can also be used at any time during the day, whenever you get a chance to relax.

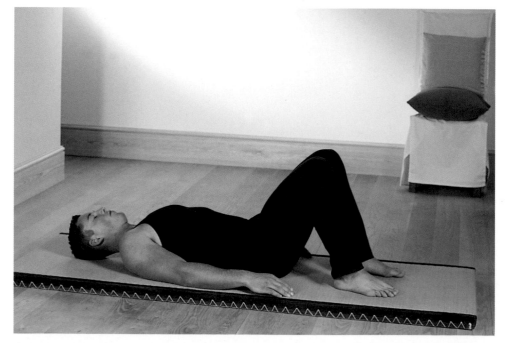

△ Lie on your back with your knees bent and your feet flat on the floor. Your spine should be in neutral. Relax your shoulders and let your shoulder blades gently glide down your spine, but do not force them into position. Your head should be in alignment with your spine and your arms relaxed by your sides. Breathe wide and full laterally, in through your nose and out through your mouth.

Exercises for mobility

During the aging process, our range of movements can decrease making everyday activities harder, increasing our risk of injuries. The following exercises guide you safely and effectively through a series of exercises that challenge mobility, so helping to keep the joints healthy and flexible. Some of the exercises also challenge your co-ordination, balance and strength.

Rolling down the spine

Now you are ready to start your Pilates session with some mobilizing exercises. This is a really effective movement for mobilizing the spine, and can be very refreshing if you have a stiff back. However, if you have problems with your spine take advice before doing it. If you find it difficult you can do it with bent knees or against the wall, and you can also keep your hands on your thighs. Keep the movement flowing and remember not to collapse into it: the abdominals should not sag. During a Pilates programme, you can use this as a transitional movement to transfer from a standing to a floor exercise, so that the feeling of flow is not lost.

Purpose: To mobilize the spine and improve balance
Target muscles: Designed to loosen/mobilize the spine
Repetitions: Repeat 6 times

Checkpoints
• Create space between each vertebra
• Bend your knees and keep your hands on your thighs if required
• Create a C-shaped spine

△ **1** Stand with your feet hip-width apart, balancing your weight evenly through your feet. Breathe in to begin and, as you exhale, lower your chin to your chest, and start to roll down towards the floor.

◁ **2** As you bend over from the hips, create a C-shape with the spine, letting the arms hang towards the floor. Feel your head relax and your shoulders drop. Don't sway backwards or forwards as you roll down. Make the movement flowing and controlled.

◁ **3** Start to curl back up, tilting the pelvis and trying to mobilize each part of the spine, uncurling it bone by bone and creating as much length as possible between the vertebrae. Try not to lean backwards or forwards but keep your weight in alignment, with your feet flat on the floor. As you come up to standing feel the crown of your head float up to the ceiling.

▷

One leg circles

Circling the legs mobilises the hip joints and also challenges core strength, as you aim to keep the hips still during movement of the lower body, your thighs get a workout too. Keep the abdominals hollowed throughout. Make sure your spine stays in neutral and your shoulder blades glide down your back. The ribs may move away from the hips in this position so keep gently reminding yourself to control them. Make the circles flow and keep the movement continuous: think of a ballet dancer's grace and poise.

FIRST POSITION

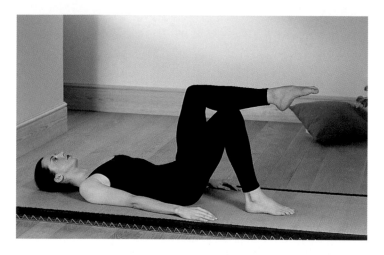

◁ Lie on your back with your knees bent and your arms by your sides. Keep your spine neutral, your head aligned and the supporting foot firmly on the floor, raise one bent leg. Ensure your hips are square and still. Then start to circle your knee. Make small circles initially then larger ones, using your abdominals for control. The breathing for this movement requires concentration: break each circle into semicircles, inhaling as your leg crosses your inner thigh and exhaling on the outer edge of the circle.

Purpose: To mobilize the hips and build core stability

Target muscles: Adductors, hip flexors and abdominals

Repetitions: Circle 5 times in each direction, then change legs and repeat

Checkpoints

• Keep the hips square: don't let them lift from the mat
• Keep the spine in neutral
• Make the circle as large as you can safely control

SECOND POSITION

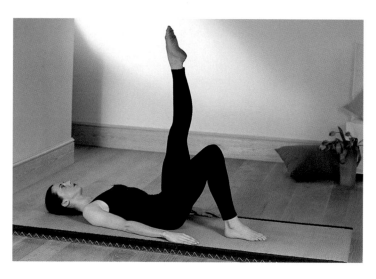

◁ Straighten the moving leg, keeping the other foot firmly on the floor. Lengthen up through your toes and try to make your leg as long as possible. If your hips start to move, you are not controlling the movement and would be better off continuing to work with a bent leg. Try to increase the size of the circle as you get stronger.

Checkpoints

• Keep the abdominals hollowed throughout the movement
• Extend the circle as you grow stronger

THIRD POSITION

◁ Straighten the supporting leg and lengthen, as if you were trying to reach the end of the room. Continue to lengthen up through the circling leg. Make the circles only as large as you can control. This position is really tough, so do not try to progress to it until you feel you have complete control in the second position. Remember to work from a strong centre.

Checkpoints

• Guard against over-curving of the spine
• Lengthen through both legs

The shoulder bridge

A very popular exercise in almost every class, this is a good mobilizer with which to start your session and a wonderful way to ease a stiff back. After this exercise your spine should feel loose and supple and it will also work your abdominals and lower body. The aim is for each bone in your spine to lift off the mat in succession. You may find that, to begin with, your back lifts in two or three sections: try to create length between each vertebra. As you lower yourself, place each vertebra in turn on the mat, imagining a pearl necklace sinking on to a velvet cloth.

The hips should be perfectly level, and you should try to create as much distance between your hips and your shoulders as possible. Do not forget to tilt the pelvis as you begin the movement. To mobilize the spine fully be sure to return to neutral as you lower your back to the floor, just before you tilt the pelvis and start the next lift.

Purpose: To mobilize the spine and challenge the abdominals
Target muscles: Erector spinae, abdominals
Repetitions: Repeat 6 times

Checkpoints
• Keep the hips level
• Maintain the distance between the hips and the ribs
• Make the movement flow

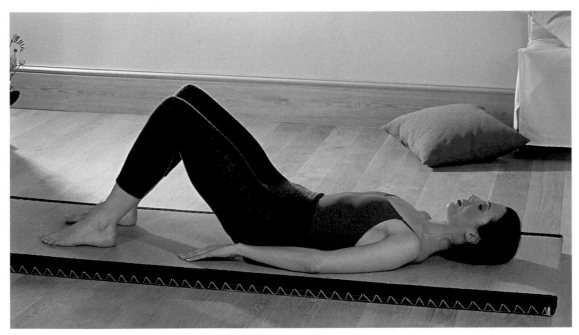

△ **1** Lie on your back with your arms by your sides, slide your shoulder blades down your spine and lengthen your arms away. Bend your knees and place your feet hip-width apart flat on the mat. Your head is in alignment and your spine in neutral.

▽ **2** Tilt your pelvis and lengthen the tailbone away. The whole length of your spine should be in contact with the mat.

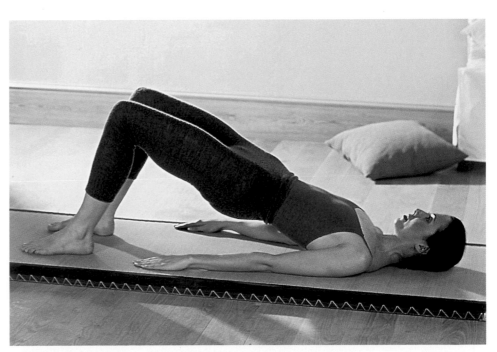

△ **3** Slowly peel your spine up off the mat bone by bone, raising your hips towards the ceiling and keeping the abdominals flat and drawn down. In this position it is common to flare the ribs, so concentrate on keeping a constant distance between the hips and ribs. Make the movement smooth and flowing, inhaling as you lift and exhaling as you come down. Once you get used to the movement you can increase the stretch by taking your arms over your head.

abdominal and back
exercises

The following exercises concentrate

mainly on the abdominals and back –

the staples of Pilates – although of course

the body works as a unit throughout every

movement. Feel the abdominals getting

stronger, flatter and firmer as you progress

and watch your wardrobe change. Your

back will respond by allowing you to live

your life in comfort and ease, free from the

burden of aches and stiffness. Pay attention

to the alignment of your body throughout

the day, for optimum results.

Rolling back

Once you have mastered this movement, it is bound to bring back memories of childhood. We all rolled back and forth when younger and it did wonders for our backs. But do remember that it may not be as effortless now that your back has stiffened up – and make sure you work on a mat that gives plenty of support. Once you have practised rolling down the spine with your hands on the floor, try progressing on to rolling back: you may not roll back up on your first attempt, but keep practising. When pulling in the abdominals, imagine you are squeezing a sponge held between your navel and your spine. Squeeze the sponge as hard as you can. Take care not to roll back on to your neck.

Purpose: To mobilize and massage the back and strengthen the abdominals
Target muscles: Erector spinae, abdominals
Repetitions: Repeat 6 times

Checkpoints
- Keep your feet flat on the floor
- Lengthen up through the spine at the end of the movement
- Tilt the pelvis

FIRST POSITION

△ **1** Sit with your spine in neutral and your knees bent with both feet flat on the floor. Place your hands near your hips with your fingers facing your feet. Inhaling wide and full through the ribs, draw your navel towards your spine. Lower your chin towards your chest then, using your hands for support, start to roll down to the floor. Try to place each vertebra on the floor, one by one. To do this, tilt your pelvis and curve your spine into a C-shape.

△ **2** Once you have rolled down as far as you find comfortable, exhale and, using your core strength, return to the starting position. Pull up through the crown of your head to create a long spine, then repeat. Use your arms only as support and avoid transferring all your weight onto your triceps.

SECOND POSITION

△ **1** Sit upright with your spine in neutral. Lengthen up through the spine and imagine your head floating up to the ceiling. Place your feet flat on the floor and your hands just below your knees. Don't overgrip: keep your elbows bent and your chest open. Take care not to tense or grip around your neck.

△ **2** Inhale as you tilt the pelvis and curve the spine into a C-shape to roll back, tucking in your chin and keeping your thighs close to your chest. As you exhale, use your abdominals to pull you back up to the starting position. Try not to use momentum, but make the movement flow at a consistent speed. Between each roll lengthen up through the spine.

Checkpoints
- Keep the chin tucked into the chest
- Do not grip the neck
- Use your abdominals to get you back to the starting position again

The roll-up

In spite of the name of this exercise, you begin by rolling down. It is an excellent way to strengthen the abdominals but is very challenging, so ensure you are comfortable and confident with the first position before moving on. Although you are curving your spine do not collapse into the movement. Roll down only a little way at first to get the feel of the movement, then roll lower as you become stronger. At all times, do a mental check that you are not tensing other parts of your body, such as your neck or face. As you come back to an upright position imagine that you are sitting against a cold steel door.

Purpose: To strengthen the abdominals

Target muscles: Abdominals, hip flexors

Repetitions: Repeat 10 times

Checkpoints

- Do not overgrip the legs, use them only as support
- Lengthen up through the spine in the starting position
- Feel the abdominals pull you up

FIRST POSITION

△ **1** Sit upright with your feet flat on the floor and your knees bent. Hold the back of your thighs, with your elbows bent and your arms open; don't overgrip. Your spine should be in neutral. Lengthen up through the spine but do not grip the neck. Slide the shoulder blades down the spine.

△ **2** Inhale and tilt your pelvis to create a C-shaped spine. Keeping your feet flat on the floor, roll down bone by bone, creating space between the vertebrae. Your hands are there to support you if you lose control but try to rely on abdominal strength to stabilize the movement. As you curl down, imagine your spine is a bicycle chain that you are placing down link by link. When you have lowered down as far as you can, exhale and contract the abdominals to roll back up to the starting position. Sit upright, keeping the spine in neutral.

SECOND POSITION

Checkpoints

- Use the abdominals, not momentum, to pull you up
- Lower bone by bone
- Do not collapse into the movement
- Keep the feet on the floor

△ **1** This time, hold your arms directly in front of you, level with your shoulders. Your elbows should be bent, arms rounded. Let your shoulder blades glide down your spine and feel the crown of your head "float" up towards the ceiling. Inhale and tilt your pelvis to begin the downward roll as before.

△ **2** When you first progress to this position try a few small roll-downs to get the feel of the movement before going down further. Feel the support of the abdominals throughout the downward and upward roll. Keep your feet flat on the floor all the time.

The hundred

This static contraction builds core strength and is one of the most commonly taught Pilates exercises. Challenge yourself to reach a hundred.

The Hundred really tests your co-ordination. Try not to stagger your breathing as you count your taps:

the breath should be flowing and even. Pay special attention to any tensing in the neck and face in this position. To help you do this exercise well, visualize a heavy weight balancing on your abdominals and pulling your navel down towards your spine.

Purpose: To strengthen core muscles, co-ordinate breathing patterns and build endurance.
Target muscles: Transverse abdominis, rectus abdominis, stabilizing mid-back muscles
Repetitions: 20 x 5 beats

FIRST POSITION

◁ Lie on your back with your knees bent, your feet flat and your head in alignment. The spine should be in neutral and the abdominals hollowed, drawing the navel to the spine. Your arms are by your sides, lifted off the mat. Slide your shoulder blades down your spine. Inhale as you count to five then exhale for five. Gently tap your fingertips on the floor and co-ordinate your breathing with your taps. Breathe steadily and laterally into your ribs.

Checkpoints
- Keep your arms lengthened
- Draw the shoulder blades down the spine
- Keep the abdominals hollowed

SECOND POSITION

◁ When you feel confident about the first position, lift your feet off the floor. Your knees should be directly above your hips and your feet level with your knees. Do not allow your knees to fall away as this will cause your spine to curve. If this is too much of a challenge you can raise just one leg, but do not twist your hips. Repeat the breathing pattern as before. Keep the abdominals flat throughout and maintain the distance between your hips and ribs.

Checkpoints
- Glide your shoulder blades down your spine
- Keep your knees above your hips
- Toes are pointed
- Feet stay level with knees

THIRD POSITION

◁ Curl your upper body off the floor, dropping your chin towards your chest so that you are facing your thighs. Do not grip your neck and keep drawing your shoulder blades down your spine. Maintain the breathing pattern for a hundred beats as before. If you want a greater challenge, try straightening the legs. Lower your eyes in this position to check that your abdominals are flat and your ribs are not flaring up.

Checkpoints
- Release tension from the neck
- Do not clench your jaw
- Keep the abdominals flat

The swimming

This exercise is a favourite with physiotherapists as it is a very effective way of developing strength in the core muscles. It is a very challenging exercise but is an easy one to cheat on, so read the instructions carefully to make sure that you are performing the exercise correctly. Ensure that you keep your abdominals lifted. Instead of just raising your arms and legs, visualize them lengthening away from your trunk. Do not try to lift them too high from the floor. Make your movements elegant and flowing and avoid throwing your arms and legs or collapsing back onto the floor on the way down. Take care not to lift your hips off the floor or to overbalance onto one side or the other.

Purpose: A strength exercise, challenging co-ordination and core strength
Target muscles: Abdominals, gluteals, erector spinae
Repetitions: Repeat 10 times

FIRST POSITION

◁ Lie on your front, placing a small pillow under your forehead to keep your head in alignment with your spine, which is in the neutral position. Keep your neck long. Stretch your arms over your head and lengthen them away. Point your toes and lengthen your legs away. Breathe laterally, wide and full. Draw in your abdominals, imagining that there is a drawing pin on the mat that you are lifting away from.

Checkpoints
• Do not tip your head back
• Keep the abdominals lifted
• Breathe laterally

SECOND POSITION

◁ Introduce a challenge to your core strength by lifting one leg. Exhale as you lift and inhale as you lower the leg. Keep both hips in contact with the floor, and do not try to lift the leg too high. Keep lengthening as you lift, maintaining the distance between the ribs and hips. Do not lose the lift in your abdominals. Take care not to twist the raised leg but keep your knee and foot in line with your hips. Repeat with the other leg.

Checkpoints:
• Lengthen as you lift the leg
• Do not twist the hips

THIRD POSITION

◁ As you exhale, lift your opposite arm and leg together. When you lift your arm raise your head and upper body with the movement, but keep facing the floor so that your head stays in line with your spine. Lengthen through your arms and legs and keep your hips in contact with the floor. Remember the drawing pin under your navel: if you lose the lift in your abdominals, continue to work in the second position for a while longer.

Checkpoints
• Keep your head in line with your spine
• Do not twist the torso
• Lengthen from a strong centre

One leg stretch

Do not be fooled into thinking that this is a relaxing leg stretch – it is actually a very challenging movement which builds core strength and is also good for improving co-ordination. Keep your hips still throughout as if they were being held in a vice. Take care not to curve your spine and keep your shoulder blades pulled down your spine and close to the back of your ribs throughout. If you find the hand position difficult, you can lightly hold either side of your knee instead. Make sure that you are just making light contact and do not over grip as this causes tension in the neck and jaw. Your upper body should be stabilized by your abdominal muscles.

Purpose: To strengthen abdominals and improve co-ordination
Target muscles: Abdominals, stabilizing back muscles
Repetitions: Repeat 10 times on each leg

Checkpoints
• Hollow your tummy throughout
• Keep the hips still

FIRST POSITION

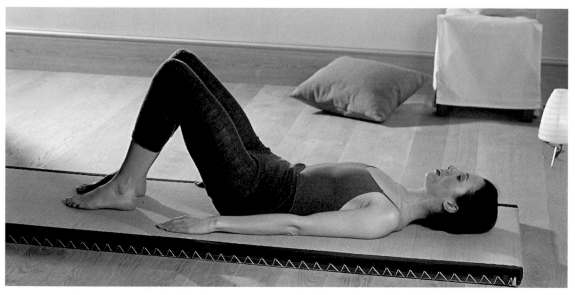

△ 1 Lie on your back with your knees bent and your feet flat on the floor. Your spine should be in neutral and your head in alignment: do not shorten your neck by tipping your head back or dropping your chin to your chest. Draw the navel to the spine.

△ 2 Lift one foot off the floor, keeping the knee bent, and pull the leg gently towards you, supporting it at the knee. Try not to overgrip, causing tension in the neck, and keep your foot in line with your knee. Take care not to let the ribs flare up. Repeat with the other leg, inhaling as you lift and exhaling as you lower.

SECOND POSITION

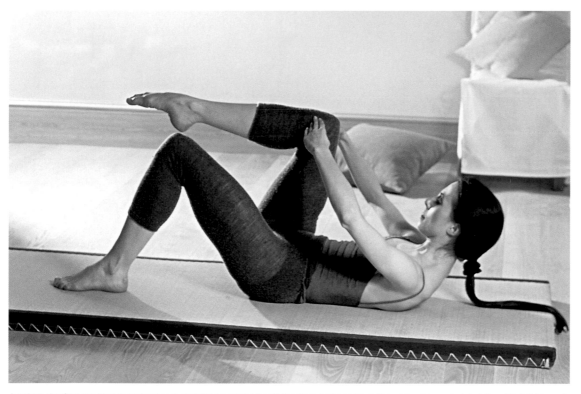

Checkpoints
- Do not tip the head forward or back
- Watch for tension in the neck

△ When the first position is understood, curl the upper body off the floor and continue the same movement. Let the chin fall towards the chest, and try to limit tension in the neck. Keep the hips very still, controlling any movement from the hips via your abdominals. Breathe laterally. Keep the stomach hollowed throughout the movement, trying to make it as flat as possible.

THIRD POSITION

Checkpoints
- Pull the shoulder blades down your spine close to the back of your ribs
- Lengthen the legs away
- The lower your straight leg, the harder your abdominals have to work

△ This position really challenges your co-ordination. As you raise the right leg, place the right hand on the ankle and the left hand on the inside of the knee. Change hands as you change legs. As one leg comes in to the body the other leg lifts and lengthens away on an exhalation. Keep your toes pointed and stretch down through the straight leg. The movement is controlled by the abdominals: keep them hollowed, and maintain the distance between the ribs and hips. Do not twist the hips: imagine they are being held in a vice. Keep the pace slow and consistent.

Leg pull prone

This is actually a yoga position as well as a modified Pilates position. You will gain a lot of torso strength and stability from this exercise, and if you do it properly it will feel as if every muscle in your body is being challenged. Remember to breathe freely throughout the exercise and do not hold your breath when holding the position. It is common to shrink down into your shoulders in this position so try to maintain the length in your neck throughout. Keep checking for tension around the neck, face and shoulders. Focus on your abdominals which should be stabilizing your whole body. You could try to visualize a drawing pin inserted through your navel and attaching to your back.

Purpose: To strengthen the abdominals and spine and challenge the upper body
Target muscles: Abdominals, stabilizing back muscles
Repetitions: Repeat up to 10 times

FIRST POSITION

◁ Lie on your front with your head in line with your spine. Bend your arms and keep your upper arms close to your body. Lift the abdominals off the floor, imagining that you are creating an arch under your stomach. Breathe wide and full. Concentrate on this abdominal lift and aim to hold it for one minute before relaxing again.

Checkpoints
• Slide your shoulders down your spine
• Keep the upper arms close to your body

SECOND POSITION

◁ Your elbows should be directly under your shoulders. Do not push your buttocks towards the ceiling or arch your spine. Keep your head in line with the spine and lengthen it away: don't sink into your shoulders or squeeze the shoulder blades together. Make sure that your hips stay square. The abdominals are lifted throughout. If this is too difficult, lower your hips and curl just your upper body off the floor. Try to hold this for one minute.

Checkpoints
• Maintain a straight line from your head to your knees
• Do not let the abdominals sag

THIRD POSITION

◁ Lift up on to your toes, straightening your legs. This is a real challenge, so be sure to have worked on the first and second positions for quite some time before progressing. Take care not to transfer all the weight into your shoulders or upper body, and keep your hips square. Pull your navel to your spine, maintaining the distance between your ribs and hips, and breathe laterally. Aim to hold for up to one minute.

Checkpoints:
• Keep a straight line from your head to your heels
• Do not transfer all your weight into your upper body
• Draw your shoulder blades down your spine

The side-kick

This is another good exercise for core strength, concentrating on the lower body. Have patience and work gradually through the progressions to achieve the best results.

When performing the Side-kick take care not to use momentum to lift and lower your leg. It may help to visualize moving your leg through mud as this will slow you down.

Your foot or knee should stay in line with your hip throughout the movement. Be aware of the alignment of your hips and keep them stacked on top of one another as it is common for the hips to roll forwards and the posture to collapse. This movement is stabilized by the abdominals and the obliques (the muscles at the side of the waist). Try to keep a constant connection with their involvement.

Purpose: To challenge core strength and work the lower body
Target muscles: Hamstrings, hip flexors, abdominals, stabilizing shoulder muscles, abductors
Repetitions: Repeat 10 times each side

Checkpoints
• Do not transfer all your weight into the arm in front
• Keep your abdominals flat

FIRST POSITION

△ 1 Lie on your side, resting your head on your outstretched lower arm. Keep your head in line with your spine, which is in neutral, and your hips stacked vertically: they must not roll in or out. Your knees are bent, one on top of the other. Place your free hand in front for balance but do not lean into the supporting arm or transfer your weight forward.

△ 2 Lift the top knee directly above the other knee. Inhale and, with your toes pointed, move the knee back as you exhale until it travels behind your body. The challenge is to keep your hips stacked and your abdominals hollowed. Your shoulder blades should be pulled down your spine and your ribs should not be pushed up. You should feel this in your side. If you want to increase the challenge straighten the top leg, keeping the toe pointed.

SECOND POSITION

Checkpoints
• Do not let the hips collapse
• Lengthen out through the legs

△ Straighten both legs. This is very challenging so be sure to advance only after working with the previous position first. Bring the bottom leg forward slightly from your hip, it should not be in line with your spine. Keep the hips vertical and lengthen out through both legs. The control comes from your centre. Exhale as the leg travels backwards.

The side-squeeze

This exercise will shape the waist and abdominals, so it is especially good for the area that hangs over your waistband when you wear fitted clothes. As you lift, check for tension in your neck or other parts of your body, and watch that your ribs stay down. Do not let the abdominals sag but hold them taut throughout.

If you wish to add an extra challenge, raise the top knee, keeping it in line with your hips – no higher. Make this a slow, controlled movement. Take care not to overgrip with your hands. Perform the movement with flow, avoiding any jerky movements when lifting and lowering.

Purpose: To strengthen the waist and mid-section, stabilizing and improving balance.
Target muscles: Obliques, shoulder stabilizers, abdominals and abductors
Repetitions: Repeat 10 times on each side

Checkpoints
- Do not allow the abdominals to sag
- Keep your hips stacked
- Maintain the distance between your ribs and hips
- Really feel the muscles in your side working

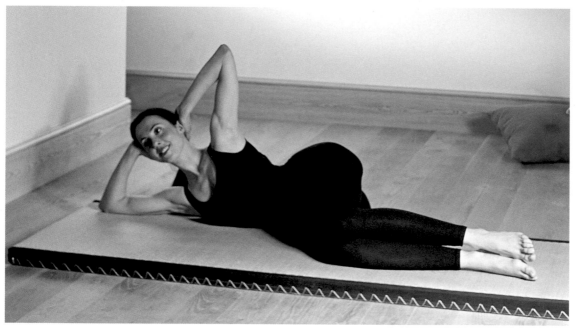

△ **1** Lie on your side with your knees bent and in line with your hips. Your hips are stacked and your abdominals hollowed. Place your hands on your head, directly opposite each other. Do not tip your head back or drop your chin to your chest. Breathe in.

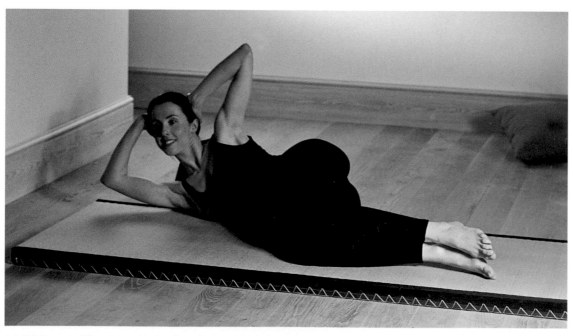

△ **2** Exhale as you lift your upper body off the floor and inhale as you lower. Make the lift slow and controlled. Don't jerk your neck or grip too hard with your hands. Maintain the length through your spine and take care not to let your hips collapse, but keep them stacked. Make sure your knees stay level with your hips. Draw your shoulder blades down your spine.

The side bend

This movement may look simple but it creates a marked improvement around the waistline if you practise it regularly, as well as developing core stability and balance. Feel the movement being controlled by your torso.

Take care in this position not to let the hips roll either inwards or outwards. Imagine that you have a red dot on your hips that should always face the ceiling as you lift. Maintain the length in your neck and avoid sinking into your shoulders. You may not be able to lift very far off the floor initially but do not worry as the real benefit comes from maintaining the correct alignment and performing the exercise accurately. You might find that this exercise is less challenging on one side than the other: it is common for one side to be a little stronger.

Purpose: To strengthen the abdominals and sides and improve balance
Target muscles: Obliques, abdominals, stabilizing shoulder muscles and latissimus dorsi
Repetitions: Repeat up to 10 times on each side

FIRST POSITION

△ **1** Lie on your side with your legs bent, knees level with hips and feet in line with knees. Imagine there is a rod running vertically through your hips. Rest on your elbow, which should be directly under your shoulder, and bring the other arm in front for support. Resist the temptation to push all your weight on to the supporting hand or the resting elbow.

△ **2** Inhale, breathing laterally, and as you exhale lift your hips off the floor. Use the muscles in the side closest to the floor to initiate the movement and control it via a strong centre. Hollow the abdominals, drawing navel to spine, slide your shoulder blades down your spine and ensure that your ribs are not pushing up.

Checkpoints
- Initiate the movement via a strong centre
- Do not transfer all your weight on to your arms
- Keep the neck soft

SECOND POSITION

Checkpoints
- Make sure the hips do not collapse
- Keep the abdominals hollowed
- Lift straight up, not veering to either side
- Keep the movement flowing

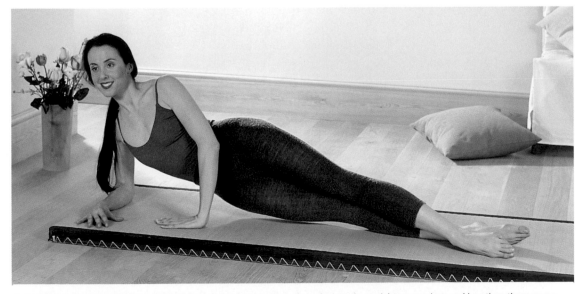

△ Progress only after reaching a level of ease in the first position. If you feel ready, straighten your legs and lengthen them away. Cross one foot over the other, with the toes pointed, to support you as you lift your hips. Keep your head in line with your spine and lengthen up through the top of your head.

upper and lower body exercises

Although Pilates is a holistic form of exercise, these movements concentrate particularly on upper and lower body strength. A number of repetitions is recommended for each exercise, but work at your own pace: if you can perform a movement accurately only twice, do so, increasing the repetitions as you grow stronger. Work your way through the progressions gradually – don't try to do too much too soon.

Push u p s

This is a classic exercise for shaping the upper body: the shoulders and biceps. If it is performed properly your abdominals will get a workout too. Once you progress beyond the first position, if your previous exercise was a standing one you can preserve the flow of movement and loosen up the spine by using a transitional move to get to the floor: follow the instructions for the mobilizing exercise called "Rolling Down the Spine" and, once your hands are hovering at floor level, bend at the knees, place your hands on the floor and move into the starting position for push-ups.

In every position, pull the abdominals in, never allowing them to sag, and keep your spine in neutral. Check for tension in your neck. Build up gradually to the full push-up.

Purpose: To strengthen the upper body
Target muscles: Deltoids, pectorals, biceps, stabilizing back muscles and abdominals
Repetitions: Repeat up to 10 times

Checkpoints
• Keep your head in line
• Do not let the abdominals sag

FIRST POSITION

◁ **1** Stand facing a wall and place your hands on it. Your hands should be level with and just wider than your chest and flat against the wall, with the fingers pointing upwards. Your feet stay flat on the floor. Keep your spine in neutral and lengthen up your body, feeling your head "float" towards the ceiling.

◁ **2** Bend at the elbows to bring your chest towards the wall. Keep your head in line with your body, slide your shoulder blades down your spine, and check that you are not pushing up your ribs. Push away from the wall to come back to your starting position. Keep the movement slow and controlled.

SECOND POSITION

Checkpoints
• Do not lock the elbows
• Lower only as far as you can control
• Keep your chest at hand level and your head forward of your hands

△ **1** Position yourself on all fours, knees directly under your hips and hands directly under your shoulders, with the fingertips facing forwards. Keep your spine in neutral and don't let your head sink into your neck.

△ **2** Keeping your head in line with your spine, exhale as you lower your chest to the floor between your hands by bending your elbows. Do not allow the abdominals to sag. As you push up, straighten the arms without locking the elbows.

THIRD POSITION

Checkpoints
- Keep a straight line from your head to your knees
- Do not let your buttocks stick up
- Do not arch or curve your back

△ **1** Drop your hips so that there is a straight line from your head to your knees. Your fingertips should be facing forwards and hands directly under the shoulders. Keep the abdominals strong and your hips square.

▷ **2** Exhale as you lower and inhale as you lift. Keep your head in line with your spine and forward of your hands. Don't let your ribs flare up. Keep your weight evenly distributed between your knees and your hands.

FOURTH POSITION

Checkpoints
- Keep your shoulder blades down the spine
- Make it a controlled, flowing movement
- Breathe laterally

△ **1** Form a straight line from your head to your feet, supporting yourself on your toes and hands. The fingertips should face forwards and your head should be in alignment with your spine.

◁ **2** Lower your chest to the floor between your hands, then push up, keeping your elbows soft. Keep the movement controlled and continuous. Lower only as far as you can control.

Tricep push ups

A common complaint is the lack of muscle tone at the back of the upper arm: this is excellent for challenging this area. It works by adapting the classic push-up to work on the triceps. The movements may look the same but there are subtle – but very important – differences. The elbows stay close to the body this time. To help you keep your elbows into your sides, visualize doing the movement in a narrow space between two walls. Try to maintain a constant, and slow, speed throughout the exercise, although this can be very difficult to maintain on the last few repetitions.

Purpose: To strengthen the upper body and the abdominals

Target muscles: Triceps, pectorals, deltoids and abdominals

Repetitions: Repeat up to 10 times

FIRST POSITION

▷ **1** Stand facing a wall. Place your hands flat against the wall, fingers pointing upwards. Your hands should be level with and just wider than your chest. Your feet stay flat on the floor. Keep your spine in neutral and slide your shoulder blades down.

▷ **2** Bend at the elbows to bring your chest towards the wall as you exhale. Unlike the classic push up your elbows should remain close to the body and pointing down at all times. Keep your head in line with your body and check that you are not pushing up your ribs. Push away from the wall to come back to your starting position.

Checkpoints
• Do not let your elbows "wing" out to the sides
• Watch for your shoulders moving up towards your ears
• Lengthen up through the top of your head

SECOND POSITION

△ **1** Position yourself on all fours, with your hands directly under your shoulders, fingertips facing forwards. Keep your spine in neutral and maintain a straight line from your head to your hips. Don't let the abdomen sag.

△ **2** Exhale as you lower your chest to the floor. This time, bend at the elbow and ensure that your elbows point towards your feet, with your upper arms staying close to your sides. As you push up, straighten the arms without locking the elbows.

Checkpoints
• Keep your chest level with your hands
• Keep your head forward of your hands
• Keep your feet flat on the floor

THIRD POSITION

▷ **1** Drop your hips so that there is a straight line from your knees to your head. Glide your shoulder blades down your spine. Your fingertips should face forwards.

Checkpoints
• Do not let your buttocks stick up
• Feel the movement in the back of your upper arms
• Do not rely on momentum

▷ **2** Exhale as you lower and inhale as you lift. Keep your head in line with your spine. Ensure that your head stays the same distance from your hands and that the elbows are pointing in the direction of your feet. Try to perform the exercise with flowing, continuous movements.

FOURTH POSITION

Checkpoints
• You should really feel this in the triceps
• Keep your body in alignment
• Hollow the abdominals
• Maintain a straight line from your head to your feet

△ Make sure you have been practising the modified positions for some time before progressing to this position. This time your whole body should be in one straight line. Don't let your head sink into your shoulders. Lower the chest to the floor, keeping your elbows pointing towards your feet and using the same breathing pattern as for the previous positions.

Tricep dips

This exercise is indispensable for firming up the muscles at the back of the arms. The tricep runs from the shoulder to the elbow and can be hard to work, but if neglected, this is the part of your arm that wobbles when you wave. Before you begin, find a chair that offers support at the correct height and check that it will not slip away from you. Work through the full range of the movement by straightening the arms, but take care not to "lock out" the elbows. Lengthen up through the top of your head.

Purpose: To tone the triceps

Target muscles: Triceps, abdominals

Repetitions: Start gently but work up to 20 times

Checkpoints
- Keep your back close to the chair
- Do not lock your elbows
- Keep your head in line

FIRST POSITION

△1 Place yourself in front of the chair with bent knees and feet flat on the floor. Support yourself on your hands with your fingers pointing forwards. Lengthen up through your spine, which is in neutral. This is your starting position. Make sure that your abdominals are hollowed throughout the exercise.

△ 2 Bend your elbows and lower your body as you inhale. Glide your shoulder blades gently down your spine and watch that your ribs do not push up. As you return to the starting position on an exhalation, take care not to "lock out" your arms, just straighten them. Keep your back close to the chair and make sure your elbows travel backwards rather than out to the sides. Execute the movement with control.

SECOND POSITION

◁ 1 Start in the same basic position as above, but this time put your legs straight out in front of you with your toes pointed. Keep your back close to the chair, your elbows pointing straight behind you and fingers pointing down. In this advanced position it is very tempting to let the elbows travel out to the sides, particularly if you are tired, or not paying full attention. Ensure that your head does not sink into your shoulders and remember to breathe fully. Your breathing should be wide and full allowing your ribs to expand fully, but keeping your abdominals hollowed out throughout the exercise. Aim to keep the movement flowing and continuous, and don't let the pace speed up or down. In this way you will work the muscle harder and get the most benefit from the exercise.

Checkpoints
- Do not use momentum
- Keep the abdominals hollowed
- Maintain an even flow

Exercises for thighs

The following exercises pay attention to the inner thighs and hips. Although you will be predominantly toning the lower body, you should still focus on hollowing out the abdominals. Ankle weights can be added to both of these exercises. Alignment is very important for these exercises so follow the directions carefully, letting the movements flow rather than "throwing" the leg.

The outer thigh blaster

If practised regularly, this exercise will really firm up the outsides of the hips and thighs and strengthen the lower body. Do not let the abdominals sag, and slide your shoulder blades gently down your spine. Maintain a constant distance between your ribs and your hips and keep the hips square, moving only your leg. Watch for tension elsewhere in the body as you do the exercise.

◁ **1** Stand facing the wall with your hands at chest level and flat against the wall. Bend one leg at the knee so that your foot is level with your knee and both knees are in line. Your spine should be in neutral and your foot flexed. Check that there is a straight line from your head to your feet, resisting the temptation to lean into the wall or bend at the hip.

◁ **2** From this starting position, take your knee out to the side. It is important to keep your foot flexed and your knees aligned. Exhale as your leg travels away from your body, inhale as you bring it back. You should not swing the leg. Don't "sink" into the supporting leg, but keep lengthening up through the spine.

Purpose: To tone the hips and lower body

Target muscles: Abductors, abdominals, adductors and hamstrings

Repetitions: Repeat 10 times with each leg

Checkpoints

- Keep your lifted foot in line with your knee
- Keep the rest of your body still; only move the working leg

The inner thigh lift

This is a popular exercise that is often done badly. However, when it is performed correctly it works wonders with that much complained about area, the inner thigh. To progress the exercise you could use ankle weights, but you should really get a feel for the inner thigh initiating the movement before moving on.

△ **1** Lie on your side, supporting your head on your outstretched arm. Your hips should be stacked and your other hand can rest in front of you on the floor for support. Bend the top leg and rest your knee on the floor. Straighten the lower leg and lengthen it away on the floor with the foot flexed. Do not curve your back or allow your ribs to jut forwards. Glide your shoulder blades down your spine.

△ **2** Inhale and, as you exhale, lift the bottom leg as high as you can, keeping the abdominals hollowed all the time, then lower it. Make the movement flow, trying to avoid any jerky movements or, worst of all, swinging your leg. You should feel the muscle of the inner thigh doing the work. Take care not to twist the knee. Keep your foot in line with your leg: there is a tendency to lead with the toes in this position.

Purpose: To tone the inner thigh

Target muscles: Adductors and abdominals

Repetitions: Repeat 10 times on each leg

Checkpoints

- Do not roll hips
- Do not curve the spine

The open V

This is not one of the most graceful-looking movements, but it works wonders for the thighs, especially the inner thighs, and also benefits the abdominals. It is very important to pay special attention to keeping your knees (and feet in the second and third positions) directly above your hips at all times. If your feet fall towards the floor, your lower back may curve upwards which could cause stress. Check that you are not holding any tension in the shoulders or neck. To create an extra challenge try placing a cushion between your knees. Of course, you won't be able to open your legs so far.

Purpose: To firm up the inner thighs

Target muscles: Adductors, hip flexors, abdominals and stabilizing back muscles

Repetitions: Repeat 10 times

Checkpoints

• Check that your feet do not drop down

• Keep your feet flexed

• Do not curve your spine

FIRST POSITION

△ **1** Lie on your back, with your knees bent and directly above your hips, and your feet level with your knees. Your feet should be flexed. Your arms are on the floor, lengthening away, your shoulder blades slide down your spine, and your head is in alignment with your spine. Start with your knees apart.

△ **2** Keeping your feet in line with your knees, bring your knees together and squeeze to feel your inner thighs working. Hold for a few seconds, then return to the starting position. Keep your abdominals hollowed throughout and your spine in neutral.

SECOND POSITION

△ **1** The basic movement is the same as before, but is done with straight legs. Lengthen up through your heels and keep your feet flexed. Start with your legs apart.

△ **2** Bring your legs together and squeeze to work your inner thighs. Keep the hips still via the abdominals, which are hollowed throughout. Keep your arms strong, and really feel your inner thighs working.

Checkpoints

- Do not allow your legs to drop away from your body
- Do not let the legs open too far
- Squeeze the knees together

THIRD POSITION

△ Curl your upper body off the floor, watching for tension in the neck and shoulders. Don't let your head sink into your shoulders, but glide your shoulder blades down your spine. Watch that your ribs do not flare up. Keep hollowing the abdominals: you can glance down and check that they are held flat. Squeeze the legs together as before.

Checkpoints

- Watch for tension in the neck
- Lengthen the arms away
- Lengthen up through the heels
- Slide your shoulder blades down your spine

Cleaning the floor

This movement will improve your balance and strengthen your lower body and all the small muscles in your feet and ankles – it is great for weak ankles. Initially, you may find the balance quite challenging. If so, it may help to look at a fixed point on the wall. It is common to find that your balance is better on one side than the other as most people favour one side. One of the objectives of this exercise is to balance any subtle differences in strength. Concentrate on maintaining the alignment between your foot and knees. If it helps, imagine that your supporting leg is held between two narrow walls.

Purpose: To strengthen lower body, feet and ankles
Target muscles: Quadriceps, supporting muscles around feet and ankles, abdominals
Repetitions: Repeat up to 10 times on each leg

Checkpoints
• Watch for your knees rolling inwards or outwards
• Keep your supporting foot flat on the floor
• Lengthen up through the spine
• Make the movement smooth and continuous

FIRST POSITION

◁ **1** Stand up tall and imagine the crown of your head floating up to the ceiling. Feel your spine lengthening. It should stay in neutral throughout. Keep your abdominals as flat as possible. Place your hands on your hips and keep your head in line with your spine. Keeping your knees in line with one another, let one foot hover above the floor as you balance evenly on the other.

◁ **2** Bend the supporting leg and lower your body as far as you can control. Do not collapse into the movement. The supporting foot may feel a little wobbly at first. Check that the knee of the supporting leg stays in alignment with the foot. Inhale as you come back up to standing. Keep your upper body strong and watch that your ribs do not travel away from your hips.

SECOND POSITION

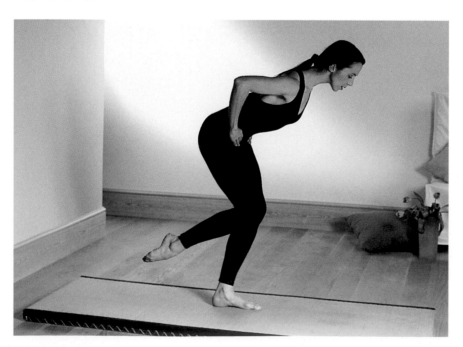

◁ Bend your knee and lower as far as you can into the position as before. This time, you are going to hold this position and then very carefully lower your chest towards the floor. Bend only a little initially. To get back to the starting position, straighten your torso first then come back up to standing. Keep your head in line.

Checkpoints
• Do not try to lower too far
• Do not collapse into the movement
• Keep lifting the abdominals

One leg kick

This core exercise really challenges your co-ordination as you cannot see the movement – you just feel it. It is fantastic for toning up the lower body while challenging core strength. A good way to visualize the movement is to imagine that you are squeezing a pillow between your hamstrings and your calf. Try to resist just placing the leg: really feel the hamstrings working. This is a deceptively hard movement so do not worry if it takes practice. You may find it easier to get a feel for the movement first, then add the correct breathing pattern and work on lengthening down through the other leg.

Purpose: To tone lower body and develop core stability and strength
Target muscles: Hamstrings, erector spinae (when upper body is lifted), abdominals, gluteals
Repetitions: Repeat 10 times with each leg

Checkpoints

- Keep the movement swift and continuous
- `Limit any movement by keeping the abdominals hollowed throughout
- Slide the shoulder blades down your spine

FIRST POSITION

△ **1** Lie on your front, supporting your forehead on your folded hands to keep your head in alignment. Draw your navel to your spine, trying to form an arch under your abdominals.

△ **2** Relax the neck. Avoid clenching the jaw. Relax your shoulders and slide the shoulder blades down your spine. Bend one leg at the knee. This is your starting position.

△ **3** Inhale and, as you exhale, point your toes and make a stabbing movement with your foot towards your buttocks. Keep your knees together and lengthen through the legs.

△ **4** Ease out of this position then repeat, this time with your foot flexed. Then extend your leg back to its original position. Meanwhile, the supporting leg on the floor should be lengthening away at all times.

SECOND POSITION

◁ Perform the same movements, but this time curl your upper body off the floor and rest on your elbows. Slide the shoulder blades down. Keep your neck long throughout and watch that your ribs do not travel away from your hips. Lengthen through the spine. If you feel a pinch in your spine in this position, stay with the first position for a while.

Checkpoints

- Keep your neck in line throughout the exercise
- Breathe wide and full
- Do not push all your weight into your arms

stretches

Throughout your Pilates sessions you will be stretching and lengthening, but here is a whole chapter to take you by the hand through one of the most popular parts of most classes – the stretches. Notice how your range of movement will re-adjust, giving you more freedom and mobility in your daily tasks. Stretching is also linked to a reduced risk of injury – something everyone can appreciate. Many people notice a distinct "lift" in their mood after stretching, feeling refreshed and invigorated, with a general sense of well-being.

Spine stretch

If your back feels tight or if you just want a healthy and mobile spine then this is the stretch for you. You will feel longer, stretched and more flexible. This is a flowing movement, not a static stretch. To keep your spine lengthening up and to stop you collapsing into the stretch, imagine that you have a beach ball in front of you, and lift up and over the ball. As you come upright again, imagine that your back is rolling up a pole, vertebra by vertebra, and take care to keep this alignment from your head to your hips: do not lean forwards or away from the imaginary pole.

Purpose: To stretch the spine

Target muscles: Erector spinae, hamstrings, adductors and abdominals

Repetitions: Repeat 10 times

Checkpoints
• Do not collapse into the stretch
• Keep the movement flowing and continuous
• Let your head float up to the ceiling

FIRST POSITION

△ **1** Sit upright with your knees bent and your feet flat on the floor. Create as much length through your spine as possible. Keep the shoulders relaxed.

△ **2** Let your chin gently drop to your chest, then roll down bone by bone through your spine. As you do so, gently reach forwards with your hands. Keep your abdominals hollowed throughout. Roll back up to the starting position and lengthen up through your spine. Do not collapse into the stretch, but lift up through the abdominals and spine. Exhale as you lower into the stretch.

SECOND POSITION

◁ The movement is the same as before, but this time straighten the legs and flex your feet, lengthening the heels away. Bend the knees slightly if you find this uncomfortable. The legs should be parted as far as is comfortable. As you roll up create as much length as possible between the vertebrae. Keep your buttocks on the floor.

Checkpoints
• Do not have the legs too far apart
• Visualize reaching up and over a beach ball
• Roll up vertebra by vertebra

Spine twist

A deceptively challenging movement, this twist will stretch the waist and lower back while strengthening the abdominals. To gain the maximum benefit, it is important to keep your bottom on the floor throughout this movement. Let your head float up to the ceiling and pull your navel towards your spine. Try to keep the movement smooth and continuous. On your first attempts at this exercise you may be surprised how hard it is to sit correctly aligned. We all develop certain postural habits and this exercise challenges them so it will feel intense at first. It gets easier with practice.

Purpose: To stretch the sides, strengthen the abdominals and promote thoracic mobility
Target muscles: Obliques, abdominals, adductors and hamstrings
Repetitions: Repeat 10 times on each side

FIRST POSITION

△ **1** Sit upright, lengthening up through the spine, with your knees bent and feet flat on the floor, legs slightly apart. Cross your arms loosely across your chest. Maintain a straight line from your head to your bottom.

△ **2** Breathing laterally, inhale and, as you exhale, turn the upper body to one side, keeping your buttocks firmly on the floor. Repeat on the other side. Remember that this is a flowing movement, not a static position.

Checkpoints
• Keep the movement flowing
• Hollow the abdominals
• Lengthen up through the spine

SECOND POSITION

◁ The basic movement is the same but is performed with straight arms, lengthening out through the arms from the shoulders. Take care not to drop them. Now you are stretching in two directions: lengthening out through your arms and up through your spine. Slide your shoulder blades gently down your back and keep your feet flat on the floor.

Checkpoints
• Do not collapse into the movement
• Keep the whole of your buttocks on the floor
• Do not curve the spine

THIRD POSITION

◁ The movement is the same but this time straighten the legs and point your toes. You are now stretching in three directions: up through your spine, out through your arms and through your legs. Be sure to keep your buttocks on the floor. You may be tempted to lean into one side as you turn.

Checkpoints
• Lengthen all the way to the toes
• Feel the abdominals working

Lower back stretch

This is a good warm-up stretch. Taking deep breaths can help you to relax into the stretch and you may find your muscles becoming more pliable, allowing you to ease yourself further into the movement. The stretch is great for easing mild tension in the lower back, which is a common complaint. Some people find it beneficial to rock slightly from side to side while in this stretch as this can gently mobilize the lower back. To do this, keep your upper body on the floor and make the movement very subtle. Although a number of repetitions are recommended, these are only a guideline until you are confident about your instincts. Hold the stretch for longer or repeat if you need to.

Purpose: To stretch the lower back

Target muscles: Erector spinae and gluteals

Repetitions: Stretch twice; hold for 30 seconds each

FIRST POSITION

◁ Lie on your back and bring both knees up towards your chest. Support your legs with your hands, just below your knees. Relax your shoulders and feel the stretch in your lower back. Remember to keep your abdominals hollowed. Inhale to prepare and exhale as you lift your legs.

Checkpoints
• Check for tension in the neck and shoulders
• Relax into the stretch
• Do not overgrip with your hands

SECOND POSITION

◁ Curl your head and shoulders off the floor, imagining curling up like a ball. Keep your neck soft: do not force your head forwards to your knees. Take care not to overgrip – keep your elbows open.

Checkpoints
• Curl up and down slowly
• Make sure your mat is thick enough to protect your back

Spine press

This movement mobilizes and stretches the lower spine. It is a good one to try whenever your lower back feels stiff, especially if you have been sitting for a long period, at your desk for example (and it can be done very discreetly). The curve of the spine should be very subtle. Take care not to over curve your spine as you may "pinch" the muscles in the lower back. If it feels uncomfortable to curve your spine, or you have problems with your lower back, you may want to perform the second part of the movement only. When you tilt your pelvis, initiate the movement by imagining you are pressing your navel towards your spine. Avoid collapsing into the movement by lengthening your spine.

Purpose: To mobilize and stretch the lower back

Target muscles: Erector spinae and abdominals

Repetitions: Stretch twice; hold for 30 seconds each

Checkpoints

• Do not overcurve your spine
• Keep the abdominals hollowed
• Keep your head in alignment

△ **1** Stand a short distance away from the wall, with your back against the wall, your knees bent and your arms by your sides. Lengthen up and glide your shoulder blades down your spine.

△ **2** Inhale and, as you exhale, push your spine flat against the wall by tilting your pelvis and contracting your abdominals. Keep your head in alignment. Try not to collapse into the movement: keep your abdominals hollowed.

Simple stretches

The following stretches are great for lengthening fatigued, tense muscles. The two upper body stretches are great for opening up the chest; this is ideal if you have been sitting at a desk for a long period of time. On the first Chest Stretch, the wrist is also being slightly stretched. If this is uncomfortable, turn your hand round so that your fingertips point to the ceiling. In the Deep Chest and Back Stretch, slightly bend your knees if your legs are stretched beyond the comfort zone. When performing the gluteals stretch, be sure to keep your bottom on the floor or you will not stretch enough.

Purpose: To stretch the chest

Target muscles: Pectorals

Repetitions: Stretch twice; hold for 30 seconds each

Checkpoints
• Keep your spine in neutral
• Feel the stretch in your chest
• Relax your shoulders

Chest stretch

This feel-good stretch is great for relieving tightness in the chest and uses the wall for support. It can be done almost anywhere to relieve tightness in the chest.

△ **1** Stand sideways to a wall. Extend one arm and place your hand flat on it. Keep your hand in line with your chest and your feet in line with your hips. Draw in your abdominals; your spine stays in neutral.

△ **2** Now turn your hips away from the wall, so that you feel a stretch in your chest. Relax your shoulders and enjoy the stretch. Change sides and repeat the movement.

Gluteals stretch

This stretch is reasonably easy to do and promotes a greater range of movement in the lower body. It is also a valuable stretch to do before many different sports that involve a lot of lower body work.

△ **1** Sit on the floor and position one leg in front of the other (the legs are not crossed). Relax your arms in front of you. Lengthen up through the spine, creating space between the vertebrae. Don't worry if your knees don't fall to the floor, just relax and let the knees fall into a natural position.

△ **2** Drop your chin towards your chest and curl down the spine while pushing the arms forwards and keeping your buttocks on the floor. Curl up again, switch the positions of the legs and repeat on the other side. Do not collapse into the movement; keep the abdominals pulled in throughout.

Purpose: To stretch the lower body
Target muscles: Gluteals
Repetitions: Stretch twice; hold for 30 seconds each

Checkpoints
- Keep your buttocks on the floor
- Replace the spine bone by bone
- Create length between the vertebrae

Deep chest and back stretch

This stretch is ideal for easing tightness in the chest and back. Try to relax your shoulders and neck into the stretch. Remember, if this stretch is too intense, you can bend your knees.

△ **1** Stand facing the wall with your feet together and place your hands flat on the wall level with your shoulders, just wider than shoulder-width apart. Lengthen up through the spine.

△ **2** Inhale, then as you exhale lower your chest by bending from the hips, to feel a stretch in your chest and back. Keep your head in line with your spine. Keep the spine lengthened and the abdominals hollowed.

Purpose: To stretch the chest and shoulders
Target muscles: Pectorals and latissimus dorsi
Repetitions: Stretch twice; hold for 30 seconds each

Checkpoints
- Keep your head in line with your spine
- Keep your hips over your knees
- Bend the knees if necessary

▷

Abdominal stretch

This is a very popular stretch that is similar to the "cobra" in yoga. It is very good for stretching the abdominals after all the hard work they have done. Take care not to throw your head back in this stretch. Keep facing the floor and lengthen up through the top of your head to avoid sinking into the shoulders. If you feel any pinching in your lower back ease gently out of the stretch.

◁ **1** Drop your hips so that there is a straight line from your knees to your head. Glide your shoulder blades down your spine. Your fingertips should face forwards.

Purpose: To stretch the abdominals

Target muscles: Abdominals

Repetitions: Stretch twice; hold for 30 seconds each

Checkpoints
• Do not overcurve your spine
• Keep your head in line with your spine
• Keep your hips on the floor

◁ **2** Inhale and, as you exhale, lift your upper body off the floor, resting the weight on your arms. Keep the abdominals hollowed and lifted, and take care not to overcurve the spine. Keep your hips on the floor. Do not sink into your neck, but lengthen up through your spine. Watch for tension in the neck. If you feel a pinch in your lower back ease out of the stretch.

Hip flexor stretch

The hip flexors tend to be one of the tightest muscle groups, and when these muscles get overly tight they can cause discomfort and eventually imbalances. People involved in most sports benefit from this stretch, especially runners.

Purpose: To stretch the hip flexors

Target muscles: Hip flexors

Repetitions: Stretch twice; hold for 30 seconds each

Checkpoints
• Take care not to collapse into the stretch
• Lunge into the stretch
• Keep your head in alignment

△ **1** Kneel down on the floor and take one step forwards, using your hands for support. If you need extra cushioning, place a pillow under the supporting knee.

△ **2** Lunge carefully into the front leg, exhaling as you lunge forwards. Make sure your raised knee is directly over your foot. Lengthen up through the spine and keep the abdominals hollowed. You should feel this stretch at the top of the rear leg. Change legs and repeat.

Waist lifts

This is a good movement to stretch and mobilize the spine. If it feels too intense or uncomfortable to have your arms overhead, then stretch with them by your side.

◁ **1** Lie on your back with your arms overhead or, if this is difficult, by your sides. Lengthen through your feet, spine and arms: visualize two cars pulling you in different directions. Draw the navel in to the spine.

Purpose: To stretch and mobilize the spine

Target muscles: Erector spinae

Repetitions: Stretch twice; hold for 30 seconds each

◁ **2** Carefully lift your waist. This is a very subtle movement; take care not to create a big curve in your spine. Keep the abdominals strong and the head in alignment. Watch for any gripping in your lower back. If you feel any pinching in your back, ease out of the stretch.

Checkpoints

• Ease out of the stretch if any pinching occurs
• Keep the abdominals strong
• Lengthen out the spine

Side stretch

This feels good at any time. No wonder cats and dogs are always stretching – it relieves the body of unwanted tension and liberates the spine and joints.

◁ Sit on the floor with one leg in front of the other (the legs are not crossed). Inhale as you prepare. Exhale as you raise one arm and lengthen up through the spine, then stretch into one side from a strong centre, taking care not to collapse into the stretch. Feel the stretch in your back. Pull the navel to the spine and keep your buttocks on the floor. If this leg positioning is uncomfortable, bend your legs and keep your feet flat on the floor.

Purpose: To stretch the back

Target muscles: The latissimus dorsi

Repetitions: Stretch twice on each side; hold for 30 seconds each

Checkpoints

• Keep your buttocks on the floor
• Lengthen up through the spine
• Don't let the abdominals sag

making
Pilates
a part of your
life

To be effective, any exercise needs to be

organized into a programme that is easy

to remember and that you will want

to do regularly. This chapter offers you

guidance on devising a Pilates programme

that will help you achieve your goals and

shows you how Pilates can become a part

of your daily life. Keep your programme

balanced. Combine it with cardiovascular

work and good nutrition to give you a

total fitness plan.

Designing a programme

With Pilates, it can be difficult to identify the muscles that are being challenged as most movements involve a combination of several muscle groups all working together. A Pilates exercise may be overtly working the arms or the legs but at the same time it may be demanding a constant stabilization process from the torso. So you will find that even though a movement is targeting a certain muscle group, you will often feel it in other parts of your body as well.

In general, Pilates movements can be divided into three main categories:

1 **Strengthening exercises** that concentrate on making certain muscle groups stronger and more toned.
2 **Flexibility exercises** that improve the range of motion around a joint.
3 **Mobility exercises** that train the body to move more easily.

◁ **Flexibility exercises will increase your range of movements and help to prevent sports injuries.**

classifying the movements

The exercises described in this book are grouped according to both the action that is being reinforced and the dominant muscles that are being used. For ease of reference, the following lists repeat this classification to help you choose a selection of movements from each group to make up a well-rounded programme. If you find an exercise listed under more than one heading it is because it involves a combination of various actions.

Exercise groups

Exercises that strengthen the upper body
- Push ups (deltoids, pectorals, biceps, abdominals and stabilizing back muscles)*
- Triceps push-ups (triceps, deltoids, abdominals and pectoral muscles)
- Leg pull prone (abdominals, stabilizing back muscles)*
- Triceps dips (triceps, abdominals)

Exercises that strengthen the lower body
- Cleaning the floor (quadriceps, supporting muscles of the feet and ankles, abdominals)
- The shoulder bridge (buttocks and abdominals)*
- The open V (adductors, abdominals, hip flexors and stabilizing back muscles)
- The outer thigh blaster (abductors, abdominals, adductors and hamstrings)
- One leg kick (hamstrings, abdominals, lower gluteals and erector spinae)*
- The inner thigh lift (adductors, abdominals)

Core exercises have been marked with an asterisk (*).

Exercises that strengthen the abdominals and back
- One leg stretch (abdominals and stabilizing back muscles)*
- The side kick (hamstrings, hip flexors, abdominals, abductors and stabilizing back muscles)*
- Leg pull, prone (abdominals and stabilizing back muscles)*
- The roll-up (abdominals, and hip flexors)*
- The side bend (obliques, abdominals, stabilizing back muscles; stretches the latissimus dorsi)*
- One leg circles (adductors, abdominals, and hip flexors)*
- The side squeeze (internal and external obliques, abdominals, shoulder stabilizers and abductors)
- The hundred (abdominals and stabilizing mid-back muscles)*
- Swimming (abdominals, gluteals and erector spinae)*

Exercises that promote flexibility
- Gluteals stretch (gluteals)
- Chest stretch (pectorals)
- Side stretch (latissimus dorsi)
- Hip flexor stretch (hip flexors)
- Spine twist (obliques, adductors and hamstrings; promotes thoracic mobility)*
- Abdominal stretch (abdominals)
- Spine stretch (erector spinae, hamstrings, adductors)*
- Deep chest and shoulder stretch (pectorals and latissimus dorsi)
- Lower back stretch (erector spinae and gluteals)
- Spine press (erector spinae)

Exercises that promote mobility
- The shoulder bridge (spine)*
- Rolling back (spine)*
- Spine twist (spine)* and Spine press (spine)
- Spine stretch (spine)*
- One leg circles (hips)*
- Rolling down the spine (spine)*

△ Consistency is one of the key elements in creating and maintaining a strong, healthy physique. Regular Pilates sessions, combined with cardiovascular exercise and healthy eating habits, will ensure positive results.

core exercises

There is an adaptation process involved in this as in any other exercise programme. This means that your body will need a few sessions to get used to the movements. You will therefore get the best results if you choose a few "core" exercises – movements that are considered pure Pilates exercises – and concentrate on these for a period of time, say four to six weeks, giving your muscles a chance to adapt to the work that is being asked of them. Start with these, and once you feel that you have mastered them (not necessarily advancing to a higher level, just feeling comfortable and confident about the movement), add on a few more.

As you add exercises, try to keep a balance between the main muscles being used: choose one from each group in turn until you have tried them all.

planning your exercise programme

How much time do you need to dedicate to your Pilates programme? How can you design a programme that will be well-rounded and complete, as well as motivating and enjoyable? When should you change the programme? What if you don't always have time to do it all? To answer these questions you need to take several factors into account.

◁ You can loosen and liberate your body with the regular practice of Pilates.

1 The time factor

In a perfect world, you would dedicate at least one hour to your Pilates programme and 30–40 minutes to a cardiovascular work-out, and you would do both activities three times a week. However, on those days when there is no time for a complete training session, a short, 25-minute workout is better than none at all.

2 Desired results

Are you trying to win a sporting event or do you just want to get a little fitter? Dramatic results require dedication, time and effort. But an hour of Pilates three times or even twice a week, as well as a weekly minimum of three cardiovascular workouts of 30–60 minutes duration, will raise your fitness level, giving you very acceptable results in a relatively short time.

3 Daily life

Do you have an active job? Do you live at the top of several flights of stairs? Do you drive everywhere or walk? The things that you do when you are not working out also count: your body does not care whether you are in a gym lifting weights or carrying a heavy box to the attic. Obviously, the more sedentary your daily life, the more conscientiously you will have to carry out your fitness plan.

Sample programmes

The majority of the exercises need to be repeated approximately ten times each (or, in the case of unilateral exercises, ten times per side). Apart from some exceptions – the Hundred is performed for one hundred taps on the mat and the Plank is held for 60-90 seconds – when putting together a programme you can safely estimate that each

movement will take about five minutes. A certain group of muscles may need more attention because of, for example, muscular imbalances or repetition of a certain activity. You also need to take into account·the initial warm-up, final stretch and a short relaxation period at the end. As an example to get you started, two basic plans are suggested here.

Vary your programme from time to time so that you do not get bored. If you dislike an exercise or it does not feel right on a particular day, do a different movement that targets the same muscle groups. Always listen to your body. Most of the exercises have variations, so work your way progressively through the different levels of intensity.

The short programme

What if you don't have time for a session lasting a whole hour? You can plan a mini programme lasting 25 minutes to do on those days when you just cannot find more time. However, do try to base most of your sessions around the hour-long plan and use the short plan only when you really have to. Twenty-five minutes is not ideal, but it's better than skipping the session entirely. Obviously, you will have to shorten the length of time spent on each exercise, as well as doing fewer of them: aim to achieve five to seven repetitions of each movement.

1

◁ **Warm-up**
8-10 minutes
(p26)

2

◁ **Push-ups**
3 minutes
(p48)

3

◁ **Swimming**
3 minutes
(p37)

4

◁ **Rolling back**
3 minutes
(p34)

5

◁ **Spine stretch**
3 minutes
(p58)

6

◁ **The Hundred**
3 minutes
(p36)

7

◁ **Relaxation**
2 minutes
(p28)

The one-hour programme

In this sample format, the exercises chosen include some of the "core" movements; this would be a good programme to start with while you are learning and adapting to these exercises. As with most Pilates programmes, the emphasis is on the strengthening of the torso.

After a few weeks, you can change some of these movements for others; try always to do some movements from each of the different categories so that you are working on all parts of the body and developing strength, flexibility and mobility.

◁ **Warm-up**
8-10 minutes
(p26)

1

◁ **The shoulder bridge**
5 minutes
(p31)

2

◁ **Swimming**
5 minutes
(p37)

3

◁ **Side squeeze: right side**
5 minutes
(p42)

4

◁ **Side squeeze: left side**
5 minutes
(p42)

5

◁ **The hundred**
5 minutes
(p36)

6

◁ **Spine stretch**
5 minutes
(p58)

7

◁ **Push-ups**
5 minutes
(p48)

8

◁ **Rolling back**
5 minutes
(p34)

9

◁ **The roll-up**
5 minutes
(p35)

10

◁ **Relaxation**
5 minutes
(p28)

11

Assessing common postural faults

The human body is a fantastic machine. It is designed to walk, run, jump, push and pull. It is autonomous and multifunctional and can adapt to many different situations - for instance, by strengthening or lengthening its muscles or adding a layer of fat to protect it from the cold. Unless you were born with a particular physical challenge, your body began life as a symmetrical and co-ordinated unit.

Unfortunately, in adult life many bodies are no longer aligned or symmetrical. The two sides function differently, with some muscles overworked and tight while others are weak and overstretched. So what does a perfectly balanced body look like? First, both sides of the body have equal strength and flexibility. The shoulders, hips and ankle joints are level and symmetrical and the shoulder blades are back and down.

posture check

Stand in front of a full-length mirror and look at your reflection. Just relax and take up your usual stance without thinking about your posture. Assess your stance honestly – or ask a trusted friend for their assessment. Here are some common misalignments of the body. Do you recognize any of these?:

- The head may be tilted to one side, jut forward or tilt backwards.
- The legs may sway backwards.
- There may be a curved "C" shape in the spine.
- The back may be over arched.
- The shoulders are not level or parallel: one may be rotated forward or elevated or both shoulders may be rounded.
- The palms of the hands are turned backwards

- The hip joints are uneven, tilted backwards or forwards or to one side
- The knees and ankles may be rolling inwards or outwards and are asymmetrical
- The feet turn in or out
- The weight is not evenly distributed between the feet
- The arches in the feet are collapsed

There are many reasons why your body has become misaligned. When any part of the body becomes dysfunctional the whole unit is affected. Even though some muscles are not doing their job effectively, you still have to get on with your day-to-day life so other muscles compensate for weaknesses. Using your body in a faulty manner reinforces these imbalances. Eventually you may start to ache in those areas that need to compensate. Aches and pains are the body's

△ The knees or ankles may roll inwards or outwards, or may be asymmetrical

△ The feet may be turned inwards or outwards

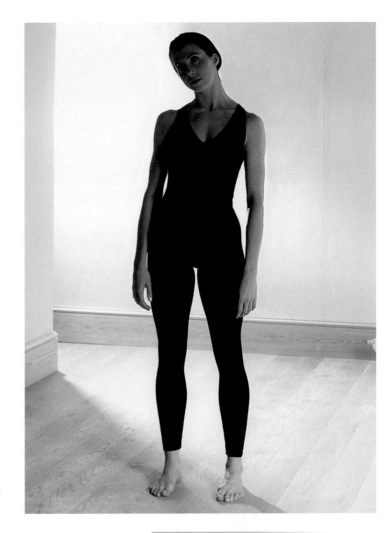

◁ The hip joints may be uneven, with the weight unevenly distributed between the feet.

▷ The head may be tilted to one side, creating muscular imbalances in the neck and back.

way of alerting you to a problem. You may even get injured or at best suffer chronic pain, commonly in the neck, back, knees, hips or shoulders. It is advisable to get an accurate assessment of the imbalance from a trained professional whilst it is still in its early stages as it is best to try to remedy the problem before your body overcompensates.

Think about the way you feel when you sit for long periods of time. Is your neck sore on one side? Does your lower back ache? This is not the way you are supposed to feel. If your body is doing its job correctly, you should not be experiencing pain or discomfort at any one place in your back or neck from sitting or standing for long periods.

So why are our bodies not doing what they were originally intended for? Most people live in a stress-filled environment. Life has become faster, more is expected, and in order to cope many devices have been designed for increased convenience and reduced effort. Devices like remote controls, lifts and cars have meant that we are less physically active than previous generations.

This lack of activity has led to a rise in obesity levels and conditions such as heart disease. We can no longer rely on general activity to keep us healthy, so we have to look at increasing our exercise levels. Stress and tension in the body can be very damaging, causing imbalances that make muscles overtight and this can lead to movement becoming restricted.

You can tell a lot about your body from your shoes. Look at a pair of your own shoes with leather (not rubber) soles. Are they more worn on the inside or the outside? Does the sole of one shoe look older than the other? Are the toes pushing against one side of only one of the shoes? Most people have slightly misaligned feet but, if this is a distinct pattern or causes discomfort, it may be worth checking with a qualified specialist. You may have an actual postural deviation that inhibits the maintenance of correct posture. If so, this should be dealt with by a medical practitioner.

▷ The head may jut forward out of alignment with the spine.

Improving your posture with Pilates

The body must be re-educated to cope with the stresses of daily life. In cases where the postural fault is severe, or there is pain, you should see a specialist before attempting this or any other exercise programme. Pilates is not meant to be an alternative to the prescription of a medical professional, but it can be a useful tool to accompany the recommendations of a specialist.

Commonly when people train in a gym they tend to choose exercises randomly, concentrating on the areas of the body they like the least, or doing exercises that they find easy to do: this can reinforce existing misalignments. Unless the body is trained as a whole, as in Pilates, its weaknesses will only be reinforced. The regular practice of Pilates strengthens and stretches all the core postural muscles, making correct posture far less of a muscular effort and more of an unconscious act.

To understand the whole picture it is essential to realize the importance of the torso. Every step you take, every weight you lift and every movement you make must be stabilized by the muscles of the abdominals and the back to protect the spinal cord against injuries. It does not matter how strong your arms are, unless your torso can protect you by stabilizing internally, your strength will be limited. Think of your body as a chain of muscles: you are only as strong as your weakest link.

If your posture is not good, your muscles will have been working in an incorrect manner for a long time. You cannot force them into place in a few sessions; there will be a period of adaptation. Always seek medical advice if you feel pain either during or after exercise. However, it is good to learn to differentiate between sore muscles and pain. Muscle soreness is par for the course

▷ When you are standing correctly, the knee and ankle joints are symmetrical and the knees face forwards.

△ The weight of the body should be equally spread between all four "corners" of the feet. Weakened muscles or rapid weight gain may have led the arches in the feet to collapse.

▷ Pilates works by strengthening the key postural muscles, making it physically more comfortable to maintain the correct alignment.

▷ Stand in front of the mirror and carefully check your posture. Pay special attention to your hips, arms, shoulders, spine and weight distribution

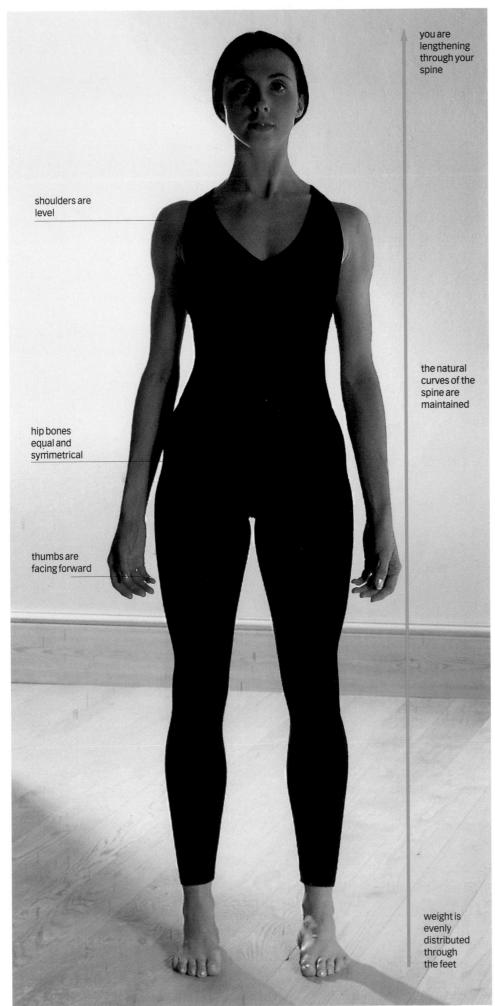

you are lengthening through your spine

shoulders are level

the natural curves of the spine are maintained

hip bones equal and symmetrical

thumbs are facing forward

weight is evenly distributed through the feet

when you begin to exercise; you will feel it most about 48 hours later. Stretching out the muscles at the end of a session helps, as can a hot bath. You may also want to try some of the wide variety of gels and creams designed to ease muscular tension. Ask your pharmacist for a recommendation.

So take up your stance in front of the mirror again. Only this time adopt what you consider to be "good posture". You should note the following points. Can you see them in your reflection?:

• Shoulders are level
• Hip bones are equal and symmetrical
• The thumb side of the hand faces forward
• The knee joints are symmetrical and face forwards
• The ankle joints are symmetrical
• The weight of the body is equally distributed between all four "corners" of the feet
• You are lengthening through your spine

▽ Become aware of how people respond more positively to you as your posture changes.

Pilates in everyday life

There would be little point in spending time exercising if you did not take a fresh look at your posture throughout the day, as you could still be reinforcing imbalances in the body that you are now dedicating time to amending. Pilates will help to strengthen and lengthen the muscles needed to maintain good posture but you also need to learn how to carry your body in the most efficient, safest way possible all the time.

posture

Your posture, the way you hold yourself, says a lot about you. When you watch someone with very good posture enter a room, observe how your eye is drawn to them and the assumptions you can find yourself making about their lives. They seem to be in control, confident and capable.

Psychologically you are also affected by your own posture: notice how much more positive and alert you feel when you sit or stand upright. Try this when making a business telephone call, it will immediately give you more confidence. Everyone is naturally more drawn to someone who seems comfortable with themselves, and research shows that we consider people with good posture to be more attractive. But most of the time you are probably unaware of the way you carry your own body; most people think about their posture only when they start getting back aches and sore necks.

▷ **Ask an honest friend to assess your posture as often we are unaware of our postural habits.**

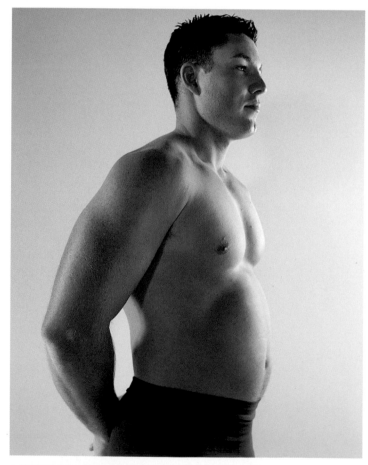

△ **Posture has a dramatic effect on our appearance. In this picture, the tone of the abdominal muscles has been completely abandoned. This lack of tone makes the model look slightly overweight.**

△ **By correcting his posture and restoring tone in the abdominals, the model looks 5-6 lbs lighter. His whole appearance has changed, presenting a slimmer and more toned physique.**

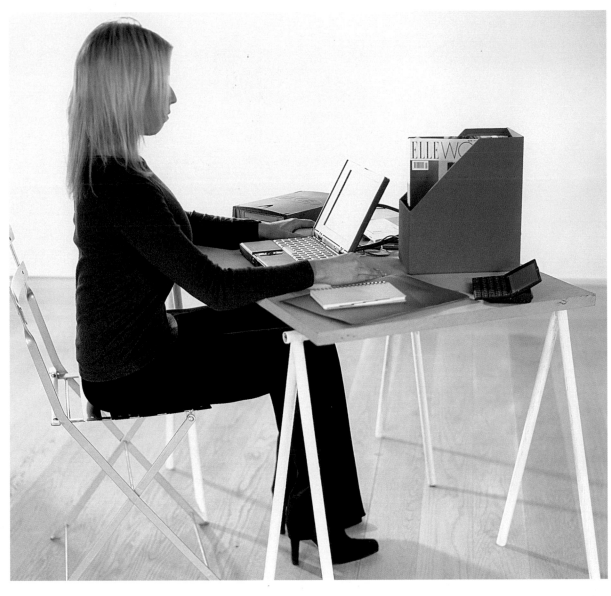

◁ Avoid flexing forward over your desk. Lengthen up through your spine with your shoulders back and down, and keep your head in alignment. Do not let the abdominals sag. Your feet should be flat on the floor, with your knees directly over them.

Posture is not just a question of how you walk or sit. To get maximum benefit from your exercise sessions, you need to get your whole body to work at maximum efficiency all the time so that it can cope with the daily demands placed on it. This means reducing imbalances throughout the body. There is little point in doing Pilates or any other form of exercise to improve your physique if you reinforce imbalances by using your body incorrectly the rest of the time.

sitting

If, like a large percentage of the population, you work in an office, you are likely to sit for long periods of time, usually in chairs that are not ergonomically correct. Practically every chair in the western world has a back rest to accommodate our slouching. In Japan, where it is common practice to sit on the floor with no support, the incidence of back pain is far lower than the estimated 80% in the West.

If you are working at a computer, writing or eating, you are likely to sit in a forward flexed position, with shoulders forward, head dropping, neck muscles tensed and spine arched. Over a period of time, this posture can become the one that you adopt every time you sit, reinforcing the muscular imbalances. It is really quite difficult to sit up straight. Your torso must be strong enough to maintain a static contraction in the back and abdominal muscles to hold your body in place. Correct alignment is the same whether you are sitting, standing or lying down: it should not change because you change positions. Whether you are standing or sitting, the shoulders should be back and down, the chest open, the abdominals contracted, the chin parallel to the floor, the feet flat on the floor.

Pilates will give you the strength to maintain correct alignment for prolonged periods of sitting. When sitting, the knees should be bent at right angles and the spine straight and lengthened but still in neutral. The legs should not be crossed. This posture can be especially difficult to maintain if you are concentrating on an activity in front of you, such as using a computer. VDU monitors that tilt and stools designed to make you sit correctly are worthwhile investments. A good way to remember your posture throughout the day is to simply write the word "posture" on your screen saver: notice the instant effect seeing the word has on you. You can also try to enrol the help of work colleagues: ask them to remind you throughout the day of your posture and to correct you if you slip into negative habits.

Whatever you are doing, stand and stretch at least once every hour. Raise your arms above your head and very gently arch and curve your back. You will feel an immediate relief in the lower back. ▷

standing

Very few people stand with their weight distributed evenly between both feet. Usually they favour one leg and then the other if they are standing for long periods of time. People with an exaggerated curve in the lower back quite often lock their knees and allow their stomachs to protrude. These habits usually result in back and knee pain. Here again, it is important to strengthen the torso in order to be able to maintain correct alignment. Refer back to the posture check and try to become aware of the way you stand throughout the day. Make a list of your natural tendencies and aim to work on one thing at a time, until you gradually adjust your habits. If it helps, tell someone close to you that you are working on your posture and get them to remind you every time they see you slump or stand on one leg.

△ When standing up, try not to favour one leg but keep your weight evenly distributed through your feet. Lengthen up through your spine with your head in alignment and your spine in neutral. Keep your shoulders relaxed.

◁ Try to avoid curving the spine and bending at the hips when lifting a heavy object.

◁ Stand close to the object, then bend at the knees and take the weight through your legs. Keep your spine in neutral with your head in alignment and keep the abdominals strong.

climbing stairs

Everyone tends to lean forward from the hips when going upstairs or walking up an incline. A certain forward flexion is normal but this should not be exaggerated as it can result in lower back pain.

When you are walking up steps or climbing a hill it is important to maintain an abdominal contraction to help stabilize the torso. Although you need to see where you are stepping, try to keep your chin parallel with the floor. Glance down at the steps with your eyes; do not lower your head.

lifting a heavy object

It is imperative to maintain stability in the torso when you are lifting anything, whether it is heavy or not. In some situations – such as catching a child who is about to fall – there is no time to prepare or brace the body for the force needed to lift an object suddenly. For this reason it is important to train the abdominal and back muscles so that they are used to contracting and the movement becomes an involuntary action.

When you do have time to prepare for the lifting of a heavy weight, bend your knees and lower the body with the torso almost erect. Place your body close to the object and use your legs, not your back, to give you the force to lift. Maintain the contraction in your abdominals the whole time, and try to lift the object from the lowest point possible. This will protect your back muscles from strain.

Exercises to do during the day

Apart from your regular Pilates sessions, there are some exercises you can do quickly and easily wherever you are. Reassess your posture throughout the day and practise the key posture points: you could even pin up a list of these and check through it from time to time. Maintaining the correct posture in your Pilates sessions helps to re-balance the body and achieve optimum results.

Drawing in the abdominals

Whenever you get the chance, practise contracting your abdominals by drawing navel to spine. This action not only tones the abdominals but will get you used to the centring movement often used in Pilates exercises.

▷ Keep your back straight and in neutral. Inhale and, imagining that you are wearing a tight pair of trousers, as you exhale pull your navel away from the waistband, making your waist smaller. Lengthen up through the spine.

Wrist circles

If you have been working on a computer it is helpful to give your wrists a stretch to make them feel looser. Remember to take a short break from your typing or writing every 20-30 minutes.

◁ Start by circling your hand. Support it with the other hand at your wrist if this feels comfortable. Circle in both directions, making a slow, full circle. Remember to keep the spine lengthened and the abdominals strong at all times.

Hand stretches

If you are working at a computer, writing or doing any other kind of repetitive movement with your hands during the day it can be beneficial to stop regularly and stretch out your hands.

◁ Keeping your hand straight and somewhat taut, draw your fingertips down towards the inside of your arm. Use the other hand to press them gently down. Now turn your hand in the other direction, drawing your fingernails towards your forearm.

Drawing the shoulder blades down the spine

This technique should be familiar from all your Pilates exercises. Standing or sitting, bring your arms to your sides with the thumbs facing forwards. Slide your shoulder blades down your spine, keeping them close to the back of the ribcage so that they are not sticking out. If you are not sure if they are sticking out or not, you can deliberately do the opposite and make your shoulder blades stick out.

▷ By gliding your shoulder blades down your spine, you will reduce the effect of any tension you are feeling in your neck and shoulders. Although hunching your shoulders up to your ears is a common reaction, it will exacerbate any discomfort you are already feeling in that area. Try to maintain the distance between your ear and shoulder at all times, unless otherwise stated. Throughout the day you can monitor the tension in your shoulders and try to become aware of situations that make them hunch up. For example, it is common for tension to increase when working at a computer for long periods of time, or when using the telephone, but by becoming aware of your habits and posture you can make a conscious and effective effort at reducing tension.

Neck stretch

When we sit for extended periods of time, especially while typing or writing, it is common to experience tension in the neck and shoulders. If you do store tension in your shoulders, it can be helpful to shrug your shoulders up to your ears, hold ... then let go. The following neck exercises will help to gently stretch and mobilize the muscles around the neck to help ease tension.

△ **1** Keeping your spine in neutral and the abdominals strong, gently tip your head, letting your chin fall down towards your chest to feel a stretch in the back of your neck.

△ **2** Turn your head slowly from side to side, taking care not to overstretch. Keep your abdominals strong and your spine in neutral.

Designing a cardiovascular programme

This book is intended to guide you through exercise in a healthy, balanced way. It deals mainly with Pilates-based exercises that will strengthen and stretch your body and give you better posture. However, in order to have a balanced programme and reach optimum fitness you also need to include exercise for the heart and lungs, known as cardiovascular exercise. There are three main components to a good fitness programme: strength work, flexibility training and cardiovascular exercise.

Cardiovascular exercise, also known as aerobic exercise, is necessary to stimulate the heart muscle. Regular cardio work will help reduce the incidence of certain diseases and will regulate blood pressure. It is also a great fat burner but this should not be your only objective.

You need to look at four important aspects of cardiovascular training when you are designing a programme: type of exercise, intensity, duration and frequency.

type of exercise

To complement your Pilates training you can choose any kind of aerobic exercise that you enjoy doing and know that you will stick with. This could be walking, jogging, cycling, swimming, hiking, aerobic dance, step - the list is endless. The main point is that you should choose something that you will do consistently. It is no good saying that you are going to make rock-climbing your main form of exercise if you live in a city and do not have the time to travel.

If you prefer company, try to get friends to exercise with you, or join a club or gym that you like and that is convenient for you to travel to. You could book in just to use the sauna or get a beauty treatment if you want to check that a gym is right for you. Try classes on offer and ask for guidance from the staff. Team sports may appeal to you, or you could combine cardiovascular exercise with a practical skill such as martial arts. Home exercise equipment is

△ **Cardiovascular exercise can be practised cheaply and effectively in the home environment. Try power walking, exercise videos or jogging. You can even dig out your skipping rope.**

widely available and need not be expensive: a skipping rope, for instance, costs very little.

Make a list of all the activities you feel you would enjoy and try them all. Cross training - doing a variety of exercise types - is advised, as the risk of injury from overuse

is less and your motivation will be kept high. You will also notice that your list will get longer as you get stronger. You will feel more capable and confident about doing different forms of activity and you will enjoy them more.

▷

intensity

How hard you should work depends on your present fitness level. The fitter you are, the more intense your workout can be, but it is important to keep the intensity of the activity suitable for your fitness level and this is sometimes difficult if you are not used to working out. It might be hard for you to distinguish between muscle fatigue and systemic tiredness. If, for example, you are cycling and your legs ache from pedalling, you may think that the exercise is very intense when really it is the weakness of your legs that is making you tired, not your heart and lungs working hard. This becomes easier to recognise over time.

During exercise, music can really help to motivate you. Try not to choose music that you brings back memories as this may distract you. Select something upbeat and positive that is not too slow.

Heart rate monitors are not essential but can be helpful in setting goals and record keeping. They are widely available and relatively inexpensive. They can also help to record recovery rates (the rate at which your heartbeat returns to normal after exercise) which document changes in fitness levels.

▽ **Aim to do cardiovascular exercise three to five times a week. There is no minimum amount of time for exercise, so if you can only manage 10 minutes it is better than none and will help to keep you motivated.**

ASSESSING EXERCISE INTENSITY

Here is a simple way of gauging the intensity of a workout. Think of a scale between 1 and 10, where 1 is no effort at all (resting) and 10 is the maximum effort that you can exert (an all-out sprint or a powerful jump). Everything else is somewhere in the middle. Remember that you are the one who subjectively puts a number to each intensity. Your number 4 might be your grandmother's number 8. Here is an example:

Mary is 38 years old, walks regularly and doesn't smoke. Her scale is:

Scale	Activity
1	Lying in bed (very, very easy)
3	Walking: 3kph/2mph (easy)
4	Walking: 5kph/3mph (getting less easy)
5	Slow jog: 7kph/4½mph (taxing)
6	Faster jog: 9.5kph/6mph (hard)
7.	Run: 10.5 kph 6½mph (harder)
8	Fast run: 12.5kph/7½mph (very hard)
10	All-out sprint: 15kph/9mph (very, very, very hard)

Simon is 55 years old, sedentary and a heavy smoker. His scale is:

Scale	Activity
1	Lying in bed (very, very easy)
3	Walking: 2kph/1¼mph (easy)
4	Walking: 3kph/2mph (getting less easy)
5	Walking: 4kph/2½mph (taxing)
6	Walking: 5kph/3mph (hard)
7	Slow jog: 7kph/4½mph (harder)
9	Faster jog: 8kph/5mph (very hard)
10	Slow run: 9 kph/5½mph (very, very hard)

What Mary perceives as being easy, Simon feels is somewhat hard, as the two are in different physical shapes.

When working aerobically, you should try to work between a four and an eight (somewhat hard to hard) on this scale. This means that the work should be a challenge, but not impossible. You should not feel as if you have been run over by a truck after your workout. If you do, you are probably working too hard. The fitter you get, the faster and harder you can work while still working between a four and an eight.

As you get fitter, you can play with this scale and sometimes may go past your last effort. This will help you to raise your threshold and prepare you for harder work with less effort. If you are out of condition, start gradually and work your way up. Do not make a heroic effort to win any races on your first day.

△ **Exercising in the fresh air makes you more alert and for those whose work is mostly indoors, being outside can help ease stress.**

▷ Joining a gym or health club may keep you motivated, but don't worry if this does not appeal to you as there are plenty of home videos available with high-standard aerobic exercise programmes for you to try.

▽ Cross training (which simply means taking part in a variety of activities) is one of the most effective ways of keeping fit. It reduces the risk of injuries, keeps you motivated and gives you the opportunity to develop a variety of muscle groups.

duration

The longer, harder and more often you exercise, the more benefits you will reap, up to a point. You will burn more fat, your lungs will become stronger, your heart will get more conditioned. However, you must start at a level at which you feel comfortable: it can be very demotivating to start off doing too much and getting injured, which could mean taking breaks in your fitness programme to recover.

The point where the disadvantages of exercise start overcoming the advantages will be different for every person. Some people have the genetics to withstand hard training, and they can make great athletes. Other people's bodies break down more easily and they should listen carefully to what their body is telling them.

Try to exercise for between 15 and 60 minutes. If you are in good shape, you can go up to the 60-minute mark. If you are just starting out, keep your workouts shorter (and less intense, of course). Remember that there is no minimum. If you can really only spare five minutes one day then this is still better than nothing.

Nothing is set in stone. Do not feel that you must exercise for unrealistically long amounts of time. Set duration goals that you will be comfortable with. It is better to

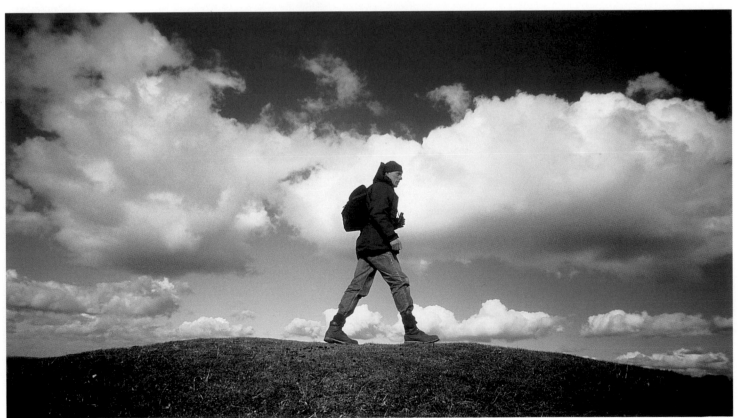

▷

do 20 minutes every other day than two bouts of 45 minutes and then never again. Obviously, the duration will be directly related to the intensity of the exercise. If you work at high intensity, you will not be able to work for very long and vice versa. Beginners should aim for longer duration with less intensity until they are strong enough to work a little harder.

frequency

How often should you do aerobic exercise? Again, you must remember that added frequency will result in greater benefits. Three to four times a week is desirable, always allowing one day of rest in between. This rest day can be active, however: you do not need to stop moving, just change what you are doing. For example, if you walk briskly on Monday you can do Pilates on Tuesday. You are resting from your cardiovascular work but it is an active rest. Consistency is a key factor in maintaining your fitness level.

To get better results, try to do aerobic exercise at least three times a week and make the rest of your life as active as possible. This could mean taking the stairs whenever you can, walking up escalators or parking the car further away from your destination, or getting off the bus a stop or two earlier. Your daytime activity does make a difference and can be classesd as exercise if it is challenging for you. Walking to or from work can be a wonderful way to relax and unwind.

If you are going to be running or power-walking, start with a warm-up then go at a gentle pace for 3-5 minutes before increasing the pace slightly, giving your body time to adjust. Here is an example of a running programme for a beginner:

△ **Cardiovascular exercise need not be boring. Dancing the night away burns up many calories.**

Week 1: Jog for 1 minute walk for 2 minutes
Week 2: Jog for 2 minutes walk for 2 minutes
Week 3: Jog for 3 minutes walk for 2 minutes
Week 4: Jog for 4 minutes walk for 2 minutes
Week 5: Jog for 5 minutes walk for 1 minute
Week 6: Jog for 6 minutes walk for 1 minute

The total amount of time you spend on this pattern will depend on how fit you are. Twenty minutes would be great but if you can only cope with 10 minutes or less, this is fine - work at your own level. Once you start you will be surprised at how quickly you can progress to jogging for 60 minutes. Carry on adding a minute week by week, decreasing your walking time, until you have reached a satisfying standard. It is important to keep setting yourself goals. Make sure you drink plenty of water before and after your run and never skimp on your warm-up or stretches as this may increase your chance of injury.

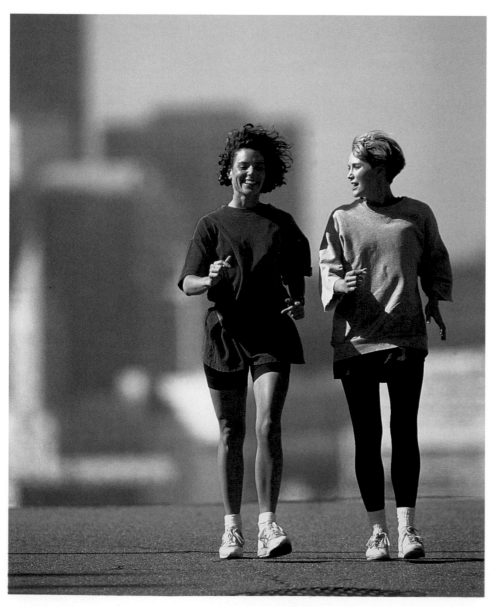

◁ **Exercising with a friend can help to keep you motivated. Make regular times to exercise and choose someone with similar objectives.**

Preparing the body for cardiovascular exercise

Warming up the body before exercise is vital to prepare it for the work that it will be asked to do. In the case of cardiovascular work you must warm up the respiratory system (heart and lungs) as well as your muscles, to help reduce the risk of injury and to focus psychologically. In a warm-up it is a good idea to simulate the exercises that will be performed during the main part of the workout, but at a much less intense level, to prepare the body gradually. As in the case of Pilates, the warm-up helps to set the mood. For cardiovascular work this needs to be faster paced: it can help to listen to upbeat music, probably slightly louder than for Pilates. When you have completed the warm-up and the stretches, start your session slowly: walk for a few minutes then build up your speed and jog. Ease your body into activity. If you begin too ambitiously you may increase your risk of injury.

The warm-up
This general warm-up could be used for jogging, power-walking (fast-paced walking), skipping or dancing. Always warm up to prepare the body for activity, both mentally and physically.

One leg circles
This mobilizing Pilates movement helps to loosen the hip joint. Work at whichever level you are accustomed to in your Pilates sessions. Repeat five times in each direction then change legs. Remember to lengthen up through your leg and keep your spine in neutral.

▷ Lying on your back, circle one leg, keeping your hips very still. Start with small circles then increase the size, controlling the movement with your abdominals.

Knee hinges
This will mobilize your knees and warm up your ankles. Keep your spine in neutral and your abdominals strong throughout the movement. Relax your shoulders and neck. Repeat five times on each leg.

△ **1** Lie on your back in the relaxation position. Lift one leg so that your thigh is at right-angles to the floor. Point your toe as you raise your foot.

△ **2** When the leg straightens flex your foot. Push your heel up towards the ceiling, then lower the foot. Think of your knee as a hinge, keeping the thigh still and limiting any movement in the hips. Exhale as you lift, inhale as you lower.

▷

Ankle circles

This will give you a wonderful loose feeling in your ankles and really wake them up. Repeat five times in each direction then change legs.

▷ Lie in the same position as for Knee Hinges, but this time rest one leg on the other. Slowly circle your ankle in one direction, then the other. Keep your toes pointed and make a full circle. Concentrate on the shape you are forming and perform this movement as slowly as you can bear. Keep your spine in neutral throughout.

Stretches

As a guide, you should hold each of these stretches for 30 seconds, but if you want to increase your flexibility or if you are particularly stiff in any area you can hold the stretch for longer. Make sure you stretch both legs equally.

Gluteals stretch

You should not only tone the buttocks but also stretch it for best effect. Stretching lengthens the muscles and may help prevent injury. Stretch before and after cardiovascular exercise for optimum effect. It is also worth timing your stretching session occasionally as it is easy to rush through it when you are tired.

Quadriceps stretch

The fronts of the thighs tend to get quite tight as you use them for most lower body activities. If they get overtight they can cause problems with the knees. The main mistake people make with this exercise is to bend at the hip, thus losing the stretch. If you find it difficult to hold your foot, loop a towel around it, and use this as an extension.

△ **1** Lying in the relaxation position, place one leg across the other, holding the supporting thigh with your hands.

△**2** Exhale as you lift the supporting leg. Keep the abdominals strong throughout. Relax your neck and shoulders and do not overgrip.

◁ Stand facing a wall or other support. Bend one leg and raise your heel towards your bottom, keeping your knees in line. Keep your abdominals hollowed. Exhale as you lift the leg. Watch for tension around the neck and shoulders, and keep your head in alignment.

Calf stretch

The calf muscles can get tight, especially if you do much walking or climb a lot of stairs.

△ Standing up with your hands on your hips, take a big step forwards. Keep your spine in neutral and lengthen up. Push the back heel into the floor to feel a stretch in the back calf. Keep the abdominals hollowed and the head in alignment. If you cannot feel the stretch take a bigger step forwards.

Adductor stretch

This is a good stretch for the inner thighs. Stretching all the muscles in the legs helps to prevent knee and spine problems.

△ From standing, take a big step out to the side. Bend one leg so that the knee is over the heel and keep the other leg very straight. Don't collapse into the stretch: watch the abdominals for sagging. Exhale as you stretch and feel the inner thigh lengthen.

Assisted hip flexor stretch

This stretch uses a chair for support, but make sure it does not slip. It is particularly good for runners, but many other people have tight hip flexors. You may feel the need to hold this stretch for longer than 30 seconds.

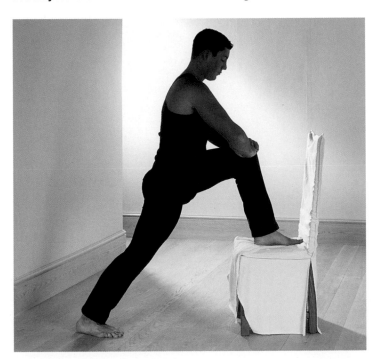

△ Stand up and rest one foot on a chair (or something lower). Bend the leg and lean into the stretch on an exhalation, keeping your back heel on the floor. Keep your head in alignment, and your spine in neutral.

Assisted hamstring stretch

This is another stretch that benefits from an additional support. The hamstrings tend to be tight in most people, and can cause back pain if left inflexible. If they do feel tight hold the stretch for slightly longer.

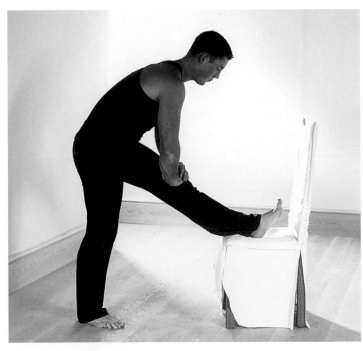

△ Standing on the floor, lift one leg and rest your foot on a support. Flex your foot and keep your leg straight, bending the supporting leg if this is more comfortable. Keep your head in alignment and your abdominals hollowed. Exhale as you ease into the stretch. Support just above the knee and try not to push down on your leg.

Nutrition: the basics

Nutrition plays a huge part in how your body performs and how you feel about it. The more you know about food, the easier it becomes to follow a sound and sane diet.

calories

People talk about how many calories there are in an apple or a piece of chocolate and they want to know how many calories they burn in exercise. But what is a calorie? One calorie is the amount of energy needed to raise the temperature of 1g water by 1°C. The same unit is used to measure the energy that food will give and the amount of energy used in activity.

nutrients

Everything you eat or drink can be included under this common heading. Your diet should consist of a balance of proteins, carbohydrates and fats, together with small quantities of the other nutrients your body needs, such as vitamins and minerals.

Proteins are most commonly found in animal products such as meat, fish and milk, but are also found in vegetables, pulses and nuts. They help the body to repair and build tissue. According to most research, if you consume up to 15% of your total amount of calories per day as protein, you will have a balanced amount in your diet. Another way to calculate this is to allow 0.75g protein per day per kilogram of your body weight.

Each gram of protein is equivalent to four calories, so if you know how many grams of protein you are eating, multiply by four to find out the number of calories. Remember that 100g/4oz of meat is not equal to 100g/4oz of protein. Meat, like most foods, consists of a number of different nutrients, as well as water, which make up the total weight. Most packaged goods will have the nutrients listed in grams as well as the total number of calories.

△ **Not all types of fat are created equally. Some fats are essential so aim to eat monounsaturated fats, found in avocados, olive oil and fish.**

The main difference between vegetable protein and animal protein is that the latter is what is called complete: that is, it contains all the essential amino acids, which are those elements the body needs to take in because it does not form them internally. Vegetable proteins (except for soya beans) are not complete unless they are intercombined (grains with beans for example), which means that vegetarians need to be careful to include the correct combinations in their diet. Try to choose low fat proteins such as chicken, fish and tofu. Limit red meat and other higher fat protein sources.

Carbohydrates are the nutrients that give you immediate energy. They are found in bread, pasta, rice and cereals as well as fruits and vegetables. You should aim to eat about 60% of your total calories in carbohydrates, but you need to differentiate between simple and complex carbohydrates. The first

▷ **Wholegrain carbohydrates are preferable to refined starches as they are richer in vitamins and minerals. They help to increase energy and provide a little protein for muscle repair. This becomes even more important when you start an exercise programme.**

(such as sugar and honey) metabolize quickly in the body and their energy is quickly "used up". The slower-metabolizing complex carbohydrates (such as pasta and rice) give you energy for longer periods of time, and at a much more even pace, maintaining a more constant blood sugar level than simple carbohydrates do.

Obviously, you should try to include more complex carbohydrates in your diet and fewer simple ones. The more refined (and usually sweet) a carbohydrate is, the simpler its composition. If possible, choose wholegrain cereals, brown rice and wholemeal pasta, which retain more of their original nutrients and also have the advantage of contributing fibre. Limit your intake of white flour, cakes and biscuits, as they tend to be high in sugar and fat. Also be aware that biscuits and cakes advertised as fat-free are not always healthier options as they can be loaded with artificial ingredients and sugar.

Fat is extremely concentrated in its energy power. One gram of fat equals nine calories; more than twice the amount of protein or carbohydrates. You need to take in fat for several reasons: it is an excellent, highly concentrated source of energy (a small amount of fat goes a long way, which was great for our ancestors but maybe not

such a prized quality today); vitamins A, D and E are stored in fat; it also makes food taste better and gives you a satisfied feeling. It is because fat tastes good that people end up eating too much of it and pumping many surplus calories into the body. Processed food manufacturers know this and add a lot of extra fat and sugar to their products to make them more appealing.

So how much fat should you consume? Most authorities agree that less than 30% of your total calories should come from fat. This may sound a lot, but almost all foods (including fruits and vegetables) contain some fat, so the calories keep piling up.

The average western diet contains around 40% fat. This, together with a lack of physical exercise, is the main reason for our spreading waistlines and the ever-increasing incidence of obesity-related illnesses. All foods will make you fat if you eat too much of them. However, fat will do the job fastest. The sum is simple: calories in (food) should equal calories out (activity). If one side of the equation does not balance the other, weight gain or weight loss occurs. All calories that are not used will be stored. However, the storage process is easier for fat

◁ Include as many vegetables as you can with each meal. There are so many different types now available that it is easy to experiment for variety.

calories than for protein or carbohydrate calories. Fat likes to end up on your body, waiting to be used on that unlikely day when there is no food to be had.

Fat is not intrinsically bad, but all fat is not created equal. Saturated fats contribute to the production of low-density lipoproteins, which cling on to the walls of your arteries, narrowing the passages and making them stiff and unpliable. The blood flows less freely and any particles that happen to be floating through can get trapped, possibly causing a heart attack or stroke. The message is to stay away from saturated fats. These are recognizable as they are almost always solid at room temperature, such as butter, lard and other animal fat. Some vegetarian products are also high in fat. Trans fats, found in margarine and some cooking oils, should be limited, as high consumption can lead to obesity and other debilitating illnesses.

Polyunsaturated fats are thought to help prevent skin complaints, heart disease and cancer. Essential fatty acids are present in fish oils, evening primrose oil, walnut oil and other polyunsaturates. Monounsaturated fats, found in olive oil, avocados, fish and nuts, are considered superior to other fats as they are linked to a decreased risk of heart disease, cancer and obesity. Most of your fat consumption should be from this last group.

Eating for life

Everyone has advice to give on eating, especially if it concerns losing weight, but very few can advise you on maintaining weight loss. Even if you find it easy to lose weight, it is very difficult to keep it off if you don't formulate a sound plan. Anyone can stick to a diet of grapefruit for a few days, or even a few weeks, but no one could or would want to maintain that kind of regime for the rest of their lives.

It can be psychologically traumatic for your weight to yo-yo. Not only must you cope with a sense of failure when you return to your average body weight, but those around you will perceive you as fighting a losing battle. It doesn't help you, but many take a great interest in other people's weight gains or losses.

When you lose weight rapidly through manipulating your diet - especially if your weight drops uncomfortably below your genetic size - and then inevitably return to your average body weight, the proportion of fat in your body may actually be higher than before. This is because some of the weight loss would normally have included lean muscle mass. Therefore you are making further problematic weight gain more likely, as lean muscle mass consumes more calories even when the body is at rest.

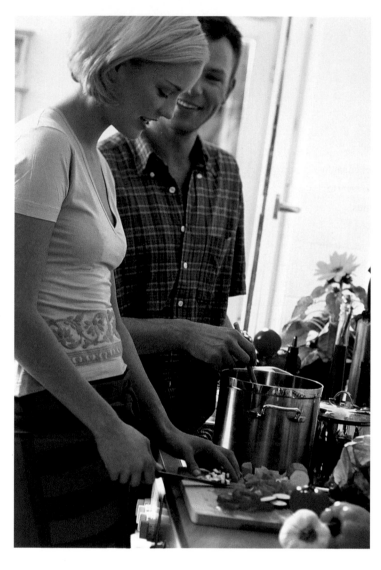

△ Try to involve your family and friends in your healthy eating habits. With their encouragement and support you are less likely to make poor choices. They may even have recipes or tips to share with you.

△ Create time to sit and eat in a relaxed manner. Eating in a hurry can lead to eating poor foods.

So what should you do if you want to lose some weight? First of all, you need to assess whether you really need to lose it. Not everyone is built like a supermodel: most bodies are designed with some extra padding, like a little warehouse ready for pregnancy or even for keeping warm in winter. No matter how hard you diet or exercise, you cannot fool your body's genetic programming. Those little fat storage areas are put there for a purpose; you may not be fond of them but they are part of your body.

This does not mean that you cannot improve your body. A sound diet and an exercise programme will make it strong. Your genes are a given but the way you treat your body will make a big difference.

maintaining your weight

The amount of calories you need to eat depends on how active you are. You want to keep fuelling your body; keep it happy and give it what it works best on. If you reduce your calorie intake too far, your body will interpret this as starvation and will react by slowing down its metabolism to save energy.

The main thing to keep in mind is that this is not a slimming diet - it is a way of eating for the rest of your life. It must be pleasurable and you must be able to lead a normal life. The plan is actually very simple: just avoid those foods that you know are high in fat and "empty calories" for most of the time and allow yourself a little more leeway for the occasional indulgence.

△ **There are so many excellent healthy-eating books on the market that it is easy to choose delicious but nutritious recipes.**

Reduce oils in your diet but do not avoid them completely. Extra virgin olive oil, for instance, is very beneficial, but fats, cheeses, and cream should be monitored. Alcohol (seven calories per gram) is another source of empty calories. This does not mean that you can never have another glass of wine: it just means that you should enjoy a glass of wine once a week instead of once a day.

Never say never again. That will only lead to frustration and anxiety. Chocolate is great, but it is very high in calories and should be enjoyed sparingly. Do not make it part of your daily diet but do not cut it out completely. If you do, you will end up dreaming about chocolate.

You should eat, and enjoy what you are eating. Food is one of the great pleasures of life. You should feel satisfied and not hungry or deprived. Think about filling up on foods that you can eat in larger quantities

UNDERSTANDING NUTRITIONAL INFORMATION

Try not to become obsessed with checking labels. Find products that taste good and satisfy your nutritional requirements, favour these then just check the labels of new foods. It can be psychologically damaging to over-analyse your diet – food should be enjoyed. Try to choose fresh, natural products, organically produced if possible. Beware of low fat processed foods as they can be full of additives, sugar and salt.

Fat

Food manufacturers may want you to believe that their products contain less fat than they really do. Take milk said to contain 2% fat. This actually means that fat makes up 2% of the total weight of the milk. But imagine a block of butter in a glass of water: if you measure fat as a fraction of weight, the butter (fat) is only a small percentage of the total. To measure the proportion of calories that come from fat, you need to know the total calories per serving and the weight of fat per serving. Take Brand X breakfast cereal:

 Total calories per serving: 378

 Grams of fat per serving: 14

There are 9 calories in a gram of fat, so 14 x 9 = 126. This is one-third of 378, so this product is 30% fat.

Calories

Calories are commonly listed in terms of serving size, which can be manipulated. The label on a chocolate bar may say it has 200 calories per portion, but there could be four portions in the bar. Some foods, such as avocados, are high in calories but also high in nutrients. Be sensible and base your choices on the percentage of fat, fibre and nutrients, rather than calories alone.

Sugar

Watch out for sugars that are not obvious, such as glucose, lactose or maltose. Of course, excessive sugar consumption not only causes dental problems but adds unwanted empty calories. A lot of fruit juices and carbonated drinks are full of sugar so try to stick to plain water for most of your daily liquid requirements.

Fibre

For a food to be classified as "high fibre" it should have a minimum of 5g of fibre per serving. Wholemeal foods, fruits, vegetables and pulses are all good sources. Fibre is important because it plays an important part in stabilizing weight and protecting against diseases such as bowel cancer.

without tipping the caloric equation. However, if you get the chocolate urge, go for it: anything else that you eat at that moment will not satisfy you. Just ask yourself if you really want to eat the whole bar or if a couple of squares would take away the

craving. Remember the 20% rule: if you only eat higher fat foods for 20% of the time you will feel less guilty. You will be surprised if you really start listening to your body. Most people in the west eat because of mental rather than physical hunger.

Make sure that you are adequately hydrated during the day: sometimes when you feel hungry you are actually thirsty. Aim to drink 2 litres/3½ pints of water a day (this can include herbal teas) as, among other things, this will give you the added bonus of healthy glowing skin. If you are going to indulge in a treat, try to eat something that has nutritional value such as nuts, rather than empty calories such as sweets.

◁ **Occasionally it is fine to eat foods that are high in fat. The key is balance. If you constantly deny yourself you will find your cravings increase.**

Frequently asked questions and answers

Will Pilates help me lose weight?

Losing weight - or rather fat - is a question of disrupting the energy balance, between calories in and calories out. A regular exercise programme will raise the body's metabolism, and although the amount of calories burnt per session may be quite small, over a period of time the average number of calories burnt will be greater. Pilates combined with a cardiovascular programme and a sensible diet will give you the results you desire.

I would like to get rid of the fat on my thighs and hips but every time I lose weight it goes from my face and breasts instead. What can I do to lose it from the right places?

Unfortunately, there is no such thing as spot-reducing. You cannot decide where you would like to remove fat, that is a decision that genetics takes for you. Many people think that by doing hundreds of abdominal exercises they will lose the fat around their middles but this is not the case. Just think about people who chew gum: if spot-reducing worked, they would have hollow cheeks! Instead of working incessantly on your lower body, you should also build up the upper body to draw attention away from the bottom half. Think what happens when you use shoulder pads - you look instantly slimmer.

I would like to start exercising again but last time I went to the gym I just got bulky and looked wider. I really dislike the current trend to be very muscular, can Pilates help?

Yes it can. Pilates builds long, lean muscles by keeping repetitions and resistance low. As it pays special attention to alignment, every move is designed to elongate as it strengthens, which is ideal for anyone who builds bulk easily. Think dancer's body rather than power-lifter's.

When will I start to see results? I have tried other programmes but I just cannot seem to stick with them long enough to see any real benefits.

If you are diligent about exercising and combine Pilates about three times a week with a cardiovascular programme and a sound diet, you should start seeing visible results within four weeks. Muscles you thought you did not have will peep through and your arms and legs will start to look more toned and streamlined. Your back will be stronger and your tummy may look flatter. However, the change won't only be visible. You will notice positive changes within yourself. You will start looking forward to your workouts and feel stronger in everything you do. You will sleep better and will most probably be in a better mood. Your aerobic sessions will become easier and you will be able to exercise for longer periods at a time. Give it a month: it's worth it.

△ Regular Pilates practice will improve your strength and flexibility.

I have quite a sway back (lordosis) and frequently experience back pain just above the kidneys. Will Pilates aggravate that situation?

Anyone with an injury or back problem should seek medical advice before starting this or any exercise programme. Pilates is an excellent technique for correcting certain postural deviations and strengthening weaknesses. However, it should not be used as a remedial method unless supervised by a trained and certified professional. Pilates will aggravate a situation such as the lordosis described above if the movements are improperly executed.

I am worried about incontinence (urine leakage) when I work out. Are there any exercises to prevent this?

The muscles of the pelvic floor can weaken, especially after giving birth. Like any other muscle, these can be strengthened to prevent the problem of incontinence. During urination, stop the flow a few times. The muscles you are using are the pelvic floor muscles and this action is exactly what you should do to strengthen them. You can do this anywhere: on a bus, at the supermarket, standing in a queue at the bank. Read the section on pelvic floor muscles for more information.

I play golf every weekend and find that I often suffer from a stiff back and neck after a game. Which exercises would be helpful in relieving or preventing this?

Pilates is an excellent training method for golfers as the customary action in this sport is quite often a hazardous one for the back. You should follow the whole programme, as all the movements will be beneficial. You may be pleasantly surprised as you discover that your game is improving with your improved strength and flexibility.

I have never exercised at all but would like to start with this programme. Could this be dangerous? I am a 54-year-old woman, slightly overweight and a non-smoker.

You should seek medical advice before starting this or any other exercise programme if you have any injuries or risk factors. These would include coronary heart disease, diabetes, high blood pressure, high cholesterol, obesity, a heavy smoking habit or a very sedentary lifestyle. Women over 50 and sedentary men over 40 should also check with their doctors.

I am extremely thin and would like to gain a little weight. What can I do? Won't Pilates just make me look even slimmer?

You probably do not get much sympathy from others as this is the opposite of most people's problem. Most bodies are genetically programmed to store fat, but yours is designed to stay very lean. Try to take in extra calories whenever you can, but do not rely on empty calories from junk food. Drink fruit juices instead of soft drinks and carry nuts and dried fruits or other high-calorie but nutritious snacks with you at all times. You should still exercise to build muscle, to give you a more toned, stronger look. Keep your cardiovascular exercise to a moderate intensity.

I cannot seem to motivate myself to exercise or change my diet. I'd like to lose some weight and get a more toned body but I lack the stimulus.

It is important to set goals that are realistic, measurable, and with a definite time frame. This will help you to look forward and stop you from seeing fitness as unattainable. You can set both long- and short-term goals. For example, "Within four weeks I want to be able to do the Hundred without having to stop halfway," is both attainable and realistic. Another motivational tool is to make a written agreement with someone who you know will support your exercise regime. Write out a contract stating that you commit yourself to exercising X times per week for X weeks. Have the other person sign as well as yourself.

◁ Although we are not suggesting that you walk around balancing a book on your head, we *are* saying that regular Pilates practice will improve both your alignment and your posture.

△ Pilates, combined with healthy eating and cardiovascular exercise, lengthens and stretches muscles creating a long, lean, strong physique.

Beware of people who may unconsciously want to sabotage your progress. Strange as it may seem, there are people who may not want you to succeed: friends who feel guilty about not taking care of themselves, mothers who are worried that you will do too much, jealous partners who worry that you will become too attractive to other people – odd, but true.

I am a single parent with no time for hobbies. I know I have to exercise but I often feel I have no free time.

When you have many demands on your time, it helps to examine all the reasons why you might choose to do something. Exercise can actually change your perspective, making you feel calmer and more in control. As they grow stronger, most people notice positive changes in their self-esteem and self-image. Headaches, backaches and depression can mysteriously disappear. With all these positive changes, exercise can become a treasured and necessary part of the day. Six weeks seems to be the point at which perspectives change. If you can reach a point where you feel you "want to" rather than "have to" exercise, it will take away the "chore" factor.

Don't forget that energy creates energy, and this will help you in your day-to-day activities. Pin up a big list of all the things that exercise will do for you, and keep it positive. For example, rather than saying "I want to be a size 10" say "I want to be confident and comfortable in my body". Do not underestimate the power of words and positive thought. Use affirmations to make you feel powerful. Sometimes it also helps to remind yourself that little is better than none at all, so start slowly and see what develops.

making Pilates a part of your life

Glossary

Bone by bone

This term refers to the movement of the vertebrae, for example in the Shoulder Bridge. As a beginner, you may lift your hips from the floor in two or three stages. As you advance try to curl up the spine, working your way up each vertebra, lengthening and straightening as you go.

Breathe laterally

This is the best way to breathe in Pilates. Breathe wide and full into the ribs, taking them out to the sides as you inhale and bringing them back together as you exhale. Avoid breathing into the stomach or high into the chest as this can also involve lifting the shoulders and chest.

Core strength

This term is given to the muscles of the torso which control all core movements in Pilates. As these muscles get stronger and your core strength increases, your posture will improve.

Control

Only work within a range of movements that you can control. Do not use momentum to increase the range. This will not work your muscles to the same extent and may cause injury. Work within your capability and progress at your own rate.

Feet flexed

This is the opposite of pointing your toes. Pull your toes back towards the shin bone.

Flow

All Pilates movements should be smooth and continuous. To help maintain flow, imagine moving through soft mud. None of the movements should be jerky.

Glide the shoulder blades down the spine

During Pilates movements you should avoid hunching your shoulders. Practise by

first hunching your shoulders up to your ears and then slide them back down your spine until you create space between your ears and your shoulders and they are at right angles to your neck. This reduces tension at the neck and shoulders. Keep them here as you exercise.

Gripping

Gripping is the unnecessary overuse of the muscles, especially around the neck, hip flexors, feet, shoulders and lower back. This creates tension in the muscles.

Hips stacked

This term refers to the alignment of the hips when you are lying on your side, for example in the Side Kick. It is common to let the hips roll inwards or outwards. The hips should be balanced one on top of the other or you may create an imbalance.

Hollow out the abdominals

This is the basis of all Pilates movements. To hollow out your abdominals, imagine pulling your navel towards your spine, as if you were wearing tight trousers and want to create space between the waistband and your tummy by using the abdominals. Do not let the abdominals sag.

Keep the neck long

This term refers to the correct position for your neck as you exercise, as well as in daily life. Try not to shorten either the front or back of the neck by dropping your chin towards your chest or tilting your head backwards, unless otherwise stated.

Lengthening

This is the opposite of shortening your muscles, which may sound obvious, but it is something that most of us do all the time without realizing. For example, to lengthen your spine imagine a balloon positioned in the centre of your head. Picture it floating up to the ceiling and try to create as much space between each vertebra in your spine as possible.

Neutral spine

This is the term given to the spine in its natural state. To check if your spine is in the correct position, flatten your back to the floor then arch it. Neutral spine is the comfortable position between the two. This position protects your spine.

Ribs flaring up

This is something to avoid. The ribs should travel out to the sides as you breathe, *see* Breathing laterally. Maintain the distance between your hips and ribs rather than letting the ribs travel up towards the chest as this often involves arching the spine.

Tilt the pelvis

This term simply means pointing the pubic bone up towards your chin eliminating the natural lumbar arch.

Transferring weight

Take care not to distribute the weight of your body unevenly, for example in the Side Bend. You may be tempted to transfer your weight on to your upper body as this is easier. Instead, rely on core strength and use the whole body as a unit.

Useful addresses

Emily Kelly can be contacted at:
Synergy
Tel: 0208 200 6055

The Global Independent Pilates
Reference Source
PO Box 19344
London
W4 1GQ
UK

The Body Control Pilates Association
17 Queensberry Mews West
South Kensington
London
SW7 2DY
UK
Tel: 0870 169 0000 (office hours)

Balanced Body
7500 14th Avenue
Suite 23
Sacramento
CA 95820-3539
USA

The Physicalmind Institute
1807 Second Street # 28
Santa Fe
New Mexico
87501
USA

The Australian Pilates Method
Association
PO Box 27
Mosman
NSW 2088
Australia

Body Studio
2/141 Wellesley Street West
Victoria Square
Auckland
New Zealand

Pilates websites are located at:
pilates.co.uk
www.bodycontrol.co.uk
www.michaelking.co.uk

Picture Acknowledgements
Superstock: 82R, 84TR, 84BL.

GettyOne Stone: pages: 81, 82L, 83T, 83B,

Author's acknowledgements

Without the help of my associates and dear friends this book would never have been more than an idea. I would like to thank Michael King and Anoushka for being great teachers; Susan Newsom, Malcolm, Tiffany, Nikki, Saban, Jeanette Haslam, and Alex Fugello; and all my wonderful clients whom I consider to be close friends. Thank you to Tanya (for being so cool), Dawn (for making me happy), Debra Mayhew, Chris Mayoral, Louise Mulryan (for making me laugh), Nicola Jones (for her extraordinary tales), my sister, Heather, my loving parents, dearest Scott and, of course, my oldest friend and soul-sister Sharon. Thank God, for all my blessings and my treasured friends.

I would like to thank Valerie Foldvary who acted as an advisor in producing this book. The following is an outline of Valerie's qualifications and experience: Valerie Foldvary has been a respected member of the fitness industry for over fifteen

years. She is a Reebok Master Trainer as well as an AFAA consultant. She holds certifications from ACE (American College of Exercise), AFAA (Aerobics and Fitness Association of America), ACSM (American College of Sports Medicine) for group exercise. She is a certified Personal Trainer and Lifestyle and Weight Management Counsellor and has also been a member of the educational committee for the revision of the ACE certification examinations for International markets.

Valerie, although of American nationality, lives in Madrid, Spain where she runs her own fitness consulting company, Californian Fitness Consultants. She writes fitness-related articles for several national magazines and has her own section on a weekly radio show dealing with health and fitness.

Valerie has been practising and teaching Pilates for several years. She conducts workshops for fitness professionals in both Spanish and English all over the world.

Index